First Talk

A Teen
Pregnancy
Prevention
Dialogue
Among
Latinos

Bronwyn Mayden
Wendy Castro
Megan Annitto

CWLA Press • *Washington DC*

CWLA Press is an imprint of the Child Welfare League of America. The Child Welfare League of America (CWLA), the nation's oldest and largest membership-based child welfare organization, is committed to engaging all Americans in promoting the well-being of children and protecting every child from harm.

CHILD WELFARE LEAGUE OF AMERICA, INC.
440 First Street, NW, Third Floor, Washington, DC 20001-2085
E-mail: books@cwla.org

CURRENT PRINTING (last digit)
10 9 8 7 6 5 4 3 2 1

Cover design by Jennifer R. Geanakos

Printed in the United States of America

ISBN # 0–87868-761-0

First Talk: A Teen Pregnancy Prevention Dialogue Among Latinos was prepared with the generous support of the National Florence Crittenton Mission Foundation, the Annie E. Casey Foundation, and the Carnegie Corporation. The views expressed in this book are those of the Child Welfare League of America and the National Council of Latino Executives and do not necessarily constitute the position of the funding organizations.

Contents

Foreword v

1. Introduction 1

2. Characteristics of the Latino Population 5

3. Factors Contributing to Latino Adolescent Pregnancy ... 15

4. Sexual Activity, Contraceptive Use, and
   Sexually Transmitted Diseases 25

5. Marriage and Childbearing 33

6. Approaches to Adolescent Pregnancy Prevention 41

7. Policy Issues 55

8. Latino Adolescent Pregnancy Prevention 75

9. Conclusion 83

Appendix A: Principles Underlying Program
   Development 85

Appendix B: Focus Groups 87

Appendix C: Participants in the Latino Adolescent
   Pregnancy Symposium 93

Appendix D: Resources 97

For More Information 105

Figures

Figure 1. Percentage Distribution of U.S. Children Under
Age 18 by Race and Latino Origin, 1980-97, and
Projected 1998-2020 7

Figure 2. Percentage of Adults Ages 18 to 24 Who Have
Completed High School by Race and Latino Origin,
1980-96 19

Figure 3. Birth Rate for Females Ages 15 to 17 by Race
and Latino Origin, 1980-97 37

Figure 4. Percent of Teen Births That Occurred to
Unmarried Teens by Race/Ethnicity, 1996 38

Figure 5. Percent of Births to Teen Receiving Inadequate
Prenatal Care by Race/Ethnicity, 1996 38

Foreword

When statistics indicated that Latino adolescents were the largest minority group to be giving birth, the National Council of Latino Executives, a group of child welfare professionals who work to enhance the lives of Latino families and children, and the Child Welfare League of America's Florence Crittenton Division organized a symposium to begin a dialogue on this concern.

A national dialogue about Latino teenage pregnancy has been absent in policy decisions that affect the Latino adolescents of this country. Therefore, we structured the symposium to produce some recommendations for child welfare practitioners and policy-making institutions to follow.

We set out to create an environment where researchers, advocates, service providers, and Latino youth could come together and contribute their own experiences and expertise on the issue of Latino teenage pregnancy. Participants heard valuable information, some personal testimonies, and policy recommendations. But the symposium became something much greater.

First, there was an amazing cultural and intellectual richness among participants. From social workers and practitioners to university researchers and directors of agencies, all participants had important contributions to make from their perspective disciplines. Not only did they represent many different regions, but they also came from a number of ethnic/cultural backgrounds that make up the Latino community. This is important, because each group of Latinos has its own set of experiences: reasons for migration to the United States, ethnic/racial mix from the country of origin, religion, etc. Having a good cross-representation from different Latino communities enabled us to speak about Latino teenage pregnancy in a way that was not monolithic, but rather, could take into consideration both our commonalities and our differences.

Second, we could not begin to discuss these viewpoints without first acknowledging that Latino teenage pregnancy is a complicated issue that threatens our children. I hope that this report has captured the quality and depth of the dialogue we experienced during the symposium.

One example of the complicated nature of our dialogue has to do with the issue of parental consent for Latinas to obtain family planning services—giving Latina adolescents access to abortions and other family planning services, without the consent of a parent, goes against the Latino value of close families. Participants struggled with the problem of how to create policy that observes and respects Latino traditional values, but also acknowledges that our children must have access to protection from HIV/AIDS and other sexually transmitted diseases.

You can see that our symposium examined conflicts and concerns that are not easily addressed, much less articulated, in current policy initiatives. This symposium is a beginning—thus, the title of our report: *First Talk*. Although there are no immediate solutions, we are finding a common Latino voice that will contribute directly to the decisions that affect our youth. In sharing our report and recommendations, we hope that many more people will engage in this critical dialogue within their own communities.

Elba Montalvo, President
National Council of Latino Executives

1. Introduction

Maria is a 13-year-old girl who is pregnant.

José is a 15-year-old teenage father.

Adrienne is a 18-year-old with two children.

Joe is a divorced 19-year-old.

Janet is a 17-year-old mother with a child on TANF.

Despite a 20-year low in the teen pregnancy rate, the United States has the highest teen pregnancy rate of any industrialized country: approximately 1 million teenage pregnancies occur annually in the United States. In spite of decreases in the adolescent childbearing rates among whites and African Americans, adolescent childbearing rates are still extremely high among Latinos (people of Mexican, Puerto Rican, Central or South American, and Cuban descent). The Latino adolescent birth rate is twice that of the white adolescent, continuing a pattern observed for many years. And for the first time, the Latino adolescent birth rate has surpassed that of the African American adolescent.

Early childbearing among Latinos appears to be strongly related to limited life options. Young women with below average basic academic skills, who come from families with incomes below the poverty level are about five times more likely to be teenage mothers than those with solid skills and above average family incomes. Latina adolescents are twice as likely than whites to give birth and are *less* likely to be informed about human sexuality and birth control and to have used contraceptives during intercourse. Latina adolescents are also *more* likely to drop out and not complete school, and more likely to be poor. These factors—and the impact of discrimination that has denied Latinos equal access to education, employment, and health care, coupled with the larger society's ignorance of the Latino culture, language, and intergenerational differences—have limited life options for Latino youth. The prosperity and progressivism of the United States are not reflected in the high incidence of the Latino adolescent childbearing rates and the low level of public and private response.

Latinos constitute one of the fastest growing ethnic minorities in the United States, with a resident population of nearly 30 million. By the year 2050, whites will become a minority, African Americans will be surpassed by Latinos as the largest ethnic group, and Asian Americans will not be far behind.* The Latino population residing in the United States is concentrated in California, New York, Texas, and Florida—states that are considered political powerhouses and that set trends for the country.

In response to these challenges, the Child Welfare League of America's Florence Crittenton Division and the National Council of Latino Executives jointly sponsored an invitational symposium (held in November 1998 and January 1999) for researchers, program administrators, and policy experts to examine adolescent pregnancy prevention in the Latino community. Symposium participants examined several key issues:

- what is known about adolescent pregnancy and childbearing in the Latino community,

---

*   F. Chideya. (1999). *The color of our future*. New York: William Morrow & Co.

- what is known about the types of programs, services, and organizations that make a difference,
- the impact of reproductive health policy on the Latino community, and
- strategies by which researcher knowledge and practitioner experience can be integrated to improve the design and evaluation of adolescent pregnancy prevention programs in the Latino community.

Participants spent a considerable amount of time discussing the gaps in knowledge, and those concerns are included in this issue brief.

Latino Youth Perspective

A total of 27 practitioners, including youth, participated in the two symposiums that yielded this report.

The importance of involving youth in pregnancy prevention efforts can not be stressed enough, so it would only be appropriate that several Latino youth were invited to participate in the discussions that lead up to this project. It is their voices and their opinions that often are missing from programs and policies designed to reach the Latino youth population.

Walton High School, located in the Fordham section of the Bronx in New York, is attended by a predominantly Latino population. The students invited to participate in the symposium were selected through the CAPS (Community Achievement Program in the Schools) program. Through this program, the Committee for Hispanic Children and Families, a New York City community-based organization, provides counseling, leadership development, and culturally affirmative activities to students identified by the school.

- David, a senior at Walton, has been accepted into University of California at Berkeley, where he intends to major in business. While he has some work experience, he is concentrating his energy on his studies.

- Mindy is a senior and is only one class away from graduation. She is currently working in a clothing store and plans to attend college and become a lawyer. She is the mother of a 2-year-old child.

- Patsy is also a senior and works for the Board of Education in New York City, School District 75. She had previously gained work experience by volunteering in a community-based organization. She plans to attend a two-year college after graduating from high school.

All of the students have been sexually active since their preadolescent years and were open to sharing what they had been taught and what they wished they had known in hindsight, to help give a picture of the gaps in their information about sexuality:

- "Sex is not bad, but the consequences are."

- "I would have liked to have waited before beginning to have sex." (Mindy, teen mom, started sexual intercourse in her preteens.)

- "Because of peer pressure, sex was something that just happened."

- "Parents don't talk about sex. Kids just want to feel comfortable talking to their parents about sex. Kids just want someone to listen." (David)

- "Programs should instill morals, respect, responsibility too, because a lot of parents are too busy."

- "I plan to go to college and become a lawyer. I want my daughter to have a better life."

2. Characteristics of the Latino Population

The Latino population is the fastest growing minority in the United States. Growth rates among the Latino population not only exceed other minority groups, but also exceed the growth rate of the U.S. population as a whole.[1] If the projected growth trends continue, the Latino population will be the largest minority group in the United States, reaching a projected 96.5 million people—24.5% of the total population—by the year 2005.[2]

Several factors contribute to the fast growth rate of the Latino population:

- the abatement of immigration policies that had previously made it difficult for Latinos to enter the United States,
- high fertility rates among Latinos, and
- the large proportion of young people in the Latino population.

Changes in immigration policies since the 1960s have had a dramatic impact on the growth rate of the Latino population.[3] In the Immigration Act of 1965, restrictive quotas based on national origins for immigrants from non-European countries were abolished, opening the door for Caribbean, Mexican, and Central and South American immigrants. The 1986 Immigration Reform and Control Act contributed to an additional increase in documented Latino immigrants by allowing a large number of immigrants to be legalized. By 1997, Latinos who were foreign born accounted for 38% of the Latino population residing in the United States.[4]

Birth rates among Latinos play another important role in the increases in the population. Latinas age 15-44 have higher numbers of children than other racial and ethnic groups and are more likely to carry a birth to term. Foreign-born Latina women from all subgroups are much more likely to have a fourth or higher order birth. Additionally, surveys reveal that Latina women both desire and have larger numbers of children than African American or white women.[5]

Compared to whites and African Americans, Latinos are a young population. Approximately 35% of Latinos are under the age of 18, while only 24% of whites and 30% of African Americans are under the age of 18.[6] The number of Latino children in the United States has already surpassed that of other minority groups. Latinos have increased more rapidly than any other racial and ethnic group, growing from 9% of the child population in 1980 to 15% in 1997. In 1998, the number of Latino children was estimated to be 10.5 million—35,000 more than the number of African American children.[7] By the year 2020, an estimated 1 in 5 children living in the United States will be Latino.[8] The growth rates only further emphasize the need for organizations that serve youth to be more responsive and better prepared to meet the needs of the diverse Latino youth population in the coming century. (See Figure 1.)

Demographics

The growth rates in the Latino population will have a greater impact on some states than on others. In 1997, more than half of the Latinos in the United States lived in either California or Texas. Six states had Latino populations of more than 1 million: California, 9.9

Figure 1. Percentage Distribution of U.S. Children Under Age 18 by Race and Latino Origin, 1980-97, and Projected 1998-2020

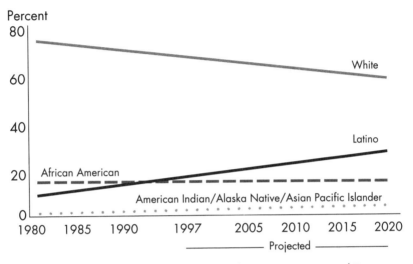

Source: U.S. Bureau of the Census, Population Estimates and Projects.

million; Texas, 5.7 million; New York, 2.6 million; Florida, 2.1 million; Illinois, 1.2 million; and Arizona, 1.0 million. California in particular has four of the ten counties in the country with the highest Latino populations: Los Angeles, Orange, San Diego, and San Bernadino. By 2025, it is estimated that the Latino population in California will grow to 43% of the total population of the state, making it the largest ethnic or racial group in California.[9] These demographic changes and fertility rates among Latino adolescents and Latina women, when coupled with the steady immigration rates, will have a profound effect on service providers and policymakers in the 21st century as they work to meet the needs of the expanding Latino community.

Racial and Ethnic Diversity

The Latino population in the United States is ethnically and racially diverse. The term *Latino* is often used in the research to include people of Mexican, Puerto Rican, Central or South American, Cuban, or other Spanish descent. In 1997, the U.S. Latino population was 63% Mexican American, 11% Puerto Rican, 4% Cuban, 14% Central and South American, and 7% other Latino origin.[10] Differences among subgroups may be more dramatic than differences between other racial groups; however, the subgroups also share many similarities. Each country's immigrants and additionally, each generation of immigrants, have come from a different level of education and economic conditions, have a different level of English proficiency, have different cultural values and traditions, and have different reasons for migration, whether political, social, or economic. Patterns of relocation in the United States, whether urban to rural, southwest to northeast, may also account for some differences in subgroups' experiences with the U.S. culture. Because of this diversity, information in this report is presented according to subgroup wherever possible. Statistical information is not often available in subgroups for Latinos, however.

Latino Culture

Latino subgroups experience a wide variety of social, political, and economic conditions that make their culture unique. Though the Latino culture is rich and distinct among the different groups, there appear to be several overarching cultural attitudes and beliefs that influence Latinos' experiences in the United States, as well as Latino adolescent development. It is important to note, however, that culture acts as an influence on behavior, not as a determinant of behavior: "Each person interacts with his or her culture in a unique way and is a complex blend of individual and cultural characteristics."[11] Although the cultural context of Latino adolescent development is crucial in understanding the conflicts and decisions that a teen may make, the cultural values discussed in this report should not be used to generalize or stereotype the Latino population as a whole.

One of the major cultural values is *familism*, which places strong emphasis on the family and children and values the traditional role of women as caretakers and mothers. Familism is commonly cited as a critical influence on Latino families and adolescent sexuality and early childbearing. Familism, however, even with the importance of the role of the woman in the family, has been shown to be a protective factor against the early initiation of sexual intercourse: "Daughters who are less acculturated are more compliant with parental traditional value systems, which act as a strong deterrent to premarital sexual behavior."[12] In addition, Flores et al. found that, among Mexican American female adolescents, those who are second generation and more acculturated engage in sexual activity early and have more sexual partners than those who are less acculturated.[13] Latinas who remain closely tied to traditional values, such as familism, may be less likely to engage in risk-taking behavior, including early or unsafe sexual activity.[14]

Another Latino cultural value that has an impact on Latino adolescent sexual relationships is the emphasis on *respeto* (respect): revering the traditional gender roles, deferring to elders (including parents and community members), and behaving in a manner that will not bring shame to the family. Marcell found that, among three generations of Mexican American males, those adolescents who adhered to traditional cultural values were more insulated from delinquent or risk-taking behavior.[15]

Latino males may also be influenced by the cultural value of *machismo*, emphasizing the traditional male role of being the family breadwinner and the traditional female role of being submissive to men.

The acculturation process is a powerful influence on the Latino population. As each individual comes into contact with the mainstream American culture, it impacts in different degrees on his or her customs, values, identity, and patterns of living: "Acculturation is a process by which people of one culture learn to adjust their behavior to accommodate the rules and expectations of another culture. The individual does not give up his or her culture in the process, but retains the identity, custom, and most everyday behaviors of his or her culture of origin."[16] Culture is dynamic and for Latino communities, cultural changes between generations can be quite extensive.[17] Latino youth are expected to learn and accept the prevailing norms from their parents, as well as the norms of the larger community that surrounds them. Many Latino youth experience the mainstream American culture more so than their parents as they progress in school. This can create a clash as they experience one culture and value set at school and a very different one at home.

The cultural norms for gender roles in Latino communities are often a powerful influence in a young person's educational attainment. Young Latinas must struggle with the pressure to fulfill the cultural expectation of becoming a mother and the desire to obtain an education. Many value the role of motherhood more than higher education, though this varies intergenerationally: "As a group, a larger percentage of foreign-born Latina teens reported their intention to be housewives and mothers as compared to U.S.-born teens."[18] Compared to African American and white adolescents, pregnant Latina adolescents reported more often that they intended to become pregnant, or that they had not been concerned about whether or not they become pregnant.[19] Latina adolescents who value both being a mother and furthering their education often end up conflicted when they become pregnant: "The more acculturated teens did not want to give up school to be full time mothers."[20]

The pregnancy rate among second and third generation American Latino teens is higher than that of first generation teens. It is believed that "foreign-born Latinas, as compared to U.S.-born Latinas, were more likely to be sexually conservative regarding the number of sexual partners and age at first intercourse. They were also more likely to have planned their pregnancies and to be married or living with a partner."[21] Researchers agree that it is important to understand the intergenerational differences in adolescent pregnancy for intervention purposes: "Fertility studies regarding Latinos have shown that fertility decreases as women become more acculturated, that is, as they increase their levels of education and speak less Spanish."[22]

Early childbearing remains an impediment to women's educational, social, and economic status in all parts of the world. Motherhood at an early age entails a risk of maternal death much greater than average, and the children of young mothers have higher levels of morbidity and mortality. For Latina young women, early motherhood can severely curtail their educational and employment opportunities with long-term adverse impacts on their, and their children's, quality of life.

With the increasing growth rates for Latinos into the next century, there is a significant need for culturally appropriate services and programs that provide Latino youth with information to empower them to have safe and healthy relationships and to lead productive lives.

Notes

1   Federal Interagency Forum on Child and Family Statistics. (1998). *America's children: Key national indicators of well-being, 1998.* Washington, DC: U.S. Government Printing Office.

2   National Council of La Raza. (1998). *Agenda Newsletter, 14*, 1.

3   Council of Economic Advisors for the President's Initiative on Race. (September 1998). *Changing America: Indicators of social and economic well-being by race and Hispanic origin.* Washington, DC: Author.

4   Council of Economic Advisors for the President's Initiative on Race 1998.

5   T. J. Mathews, S. J. Ventura, S. C. Curtin, & J. A. Martin. (1998). *Births of Hispanic origins, 1989-95.* Monthly vital statistics report, Vol. 46, No. 6, Supplement. Hyattsville, MD: National Center for Health Statistics.

6   Council of Economic Advisors for the President's Initiative on Race 1998.

7   National Council of La Raza 1998.

8   Federal Interagency Forum on Child and Family Statistics 1998.

9   National Council of La Raza 1998.

10   National Council of La Raza 1998.

11   T. Cross. (Fall/Winter 1995-96). Developing a knowledge base to support cultural competence. *Family Resource Coalition Report,* 14.

12   C. Brindis. (September 1992). Adolescent pregnancy prevention for Hispanic youth: The role of schools, families, and communities. *Journal of School Health, 67* (7), 345-351.

13 E. Flores, S. L. Eyre, & S. G. Millstein. (February 1998). Sociocultural beliefs related to sex among Mexican American adolescents. *Hispanic Journal of Behavioral Sciences*, 20 (1).

14 A. Marcell. (1994). Understanding ethnicity, identity formation, and risk behavior among adolescents of Mexican descent. *Journal of School Health, 64* (8).

15 Marcell 1994.

16 Cross 1995-96.

17 Brindis 1992.

18 J. Solis. (1995). The status of Latino children and youth: Challenges and prospects. In R. Zambrana (Ed.), *Understanding Latino families: Scholarship, policy, and practice*. Thousand Oaks, CA: Sage Publications.

19 Alan Guttmacher Institute. (1994). *Sex and America's teenagers*. New York: The Alan Guttmacher Institute.

20 Solis 1995.

21 Solis 1995; Brindis 1992; Marcell 1994.

22 F. D. Bean & G. Swicegood. (1982). Generation, female education, and Mexican American fertility. *Social Science Quarterly, 63* (1), 131-144. A. M. Sorensen. (1988). The fertility and language characteristics of Mexican-American and non-Hispanic husbands and wives. *The Sociological Quarterly, 29* (1), 111-130. In Solis 1995.

3. Factors Contributing to Latino Adolescent Pregnancy

A number of factors have been documented in the research as antecedents to or risk factors associated with adolescent pregnancy and premature parenthood: poverty, family dysfunction, low educational achievement, and risk-taking behaviors. For the Latino population, however, many of these risk factors impact on Latino youth in unique ways often not addressed or perhaps not even recognized by prevention programs and policymakers. This chapter will explore socioeconomic status, health care accessibility, educational attainment, religiousness, and milestones of adolescent development as they impact on adolescent pregnancy in the Latino community.

Socioeconomic Status

Research shows a direct relationship between the poverty level, education level of parents, and adolescent pregnancy rates: young people who live in extreme poverty with parents who have low levels of education have higher rates of pregnancy than youth in middle- to high-income families.[1] In fact, 80% of young women who give birth are poor.[2] Therefore, information regarding the socioeconomic status of Latino families is critical in the discussion of adolescent childbearing.

Latinos have the highest poverty rate of any major racial or ethnic group in the United States.[3] Between 1995 and 1996, the poverty rate for Latinos remained at 29.4%, higher than the poverty rate for either African Americans (28.4%) or whites (11.0%).[4] Median family income for Latinos was $26,179 in 1996, compared to $44,756 for white families, and $26,522 for African American families.[5] In 1995, 39.3% of Latino families with children under age 18 lived below the poverty level, and 57.3% of Latino families headed by a single mother with children under the age of 18 lived below the poverty level.[6] Latinos and whites have the largest numbers of children living in poverty. When the proportions are examined, however, 40% of Latino children and 40% of African American children were living in poverty, compared to only 10% of white children in 1996.[7] The decrease in socioeconomic status for the Latino population is attributed to the large numbers of Latino immigrants who often have less education and lower incomes than the Latino population as a whole.

Health Care

Latinos were more than twice as likely to lack health insurance as whites in 1995 (32% of Latinos were uninsured, compared to 13% of whites).[8] Overall, the Latino population is the most likely of all racial and ethnic groups to be uninsured or underinsured. Even though the percent of the population that is uninsured does decrease as income level increases, Latinos are most likely to have higher rates of being uninsured in all income levels when compared to whites and African Americans.[9]

As compared to white or African American children, Latino children under the age of 18 are the least likely to have health insurance.[10] For Latino adolescents, approximately 34% are uninsured, as compared to 13% of white adolescents. Subgroup data reveal that a larger percent of Mexican adolescents do not have health insurance as compared to Puerto Rican adolescents (37% to 11%, respectively).[11] This issue is of particular concern to programs that provide adolescent pregnancy prevention efforts and prenatal services for pregnant adolescents.

Another group falling through the cracks in the nation's health care system are children in undocumented Latino families. Illegal immigrants face great medical risks, for they are most likely to be living in poverty, have little access to health care and family planning services, and are most likely to have health problems.[12] Efforts to provide health care for undocumented Latino families often prove difficult, as many undocumented Latinos are wary of coming into contact with figures of authority, for fear of being reported.

Education

Latino youth make up approximately 14% of the school-age population, and by the year 2020, the census estimates that Latino youth will make up 22% of the school-age population. However, according to administrative officials, Latino advocates, and academic experts, "Those children are falling behind in school in a manner that could have a serious economic effect on the whole nation."[13]

The proportion of high school dropouts in the Latino population is significantly higher than any other major ethnic group.[14] In 1994, the dropout rate for Latinos between the ages of 16 and 24 was between 30 and 35%, compared to 12.6% among African Americans and 10.5% among whites.[15] Latinos have lower high school completion rates than either African Americans and whites, fluctuating between a low of 57% in 1980 and a high of 67% in 1985 during the 1980-1996 period.[16] The Latino high school completion rate was approximately 62% in 1996.[17] Dropout rates and low educational achievement are closely associated with rates of adolescent pregnancy, making the high incidence of leaving high school among young Latinos a paramount concern.

Other troubling problems persist. Not only do Latino youth drop out of high school at twice the rate of other groups, they are also dropping out at a younger age. The percentage of Latino youth who drop out before finishing the tenth grade is 55%, compared to approximately 30% for white youth and 25% for African American youth.[18] In fact, one study from 1988 showed that, among Latino youth ages 16-24 who had not completed a high school education, at least half of the group had never even begun high school: 32% had ended their education at the sixth grade or earlier and another 34% had dropped out between the seventh and ninth grade.[19] An additional challenge for the education community is that Latino youth who drop out of high school are less likely to return to school or complete a GED.[20] (See Figure 2.)

Causes for high school dropout rates vary. Latino males frequently reported leaving school for economic reasons and the need to work. Discrimination and cultural and language barriers often precipitate Latino students leaving school, because they feel pushed out or alienated from the educational system. The majority of Latino youth attend segregated schools, with inadequate resources, fewer high-quality teachers, less rigorous classes, and lower teacher expectations for their performance than their white counterparts.[21] For Latina adolescents, low educational aspirations among peers was found to be particularly influential when reporting reasons for leaving school. Latinas were more likely than African Americans or whites to have left school before they were pregnant. Latinas are less likely to return to school after having a child, placing them at greater risk for future economic hardships. Further understanding the reasons that lead Latinas to leave school may be particularly useful in early pregnancy prevention efforts.

Figure 2. Percentage of Adults Ages 18 to 24 Who Have Completed High School by Race and Latino Origin, 1980-96

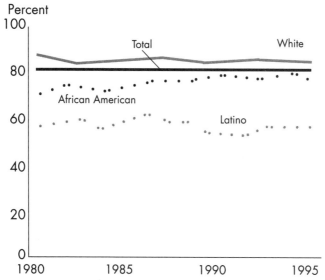

Note: Percentages are based only on those not currently enrolled in high school or below. Prior to 1992, this indicator was measured as completing four or more years of high school.
Source: U.S. Bureau of the Census, October Current Population Survey. Tabulated by the U.S. Department of Education, National Center for Education Statistics.

School connectedness, defined by adolescents in grades 7-12 as feeling close to people at school, feeling a part of the school, getting along with teachers and peers, and feeling that the teachers treat the students fairly, has been shown to be a protective factor in delaying initiation of sexual intercourse.[22] With Latino youth dropping out of school in large numbers prior to the ninth grade, the American school system is clearly failing to help Latino youth feel a sense of connectedness to their school, further placing them at greater risk for early sexual activity, unintended pregnancy, and limited life options.

Religion

Religion and spirituality play a strong role in the traditional Latino culture. Religious affiliations differ somewhat, depending on ethnicity. For instance, 96% of Mexicans are Roman Catholics, while the predominant religions among Puerto Ricans are Catholicism and Protestantism (Evangelical and Pentecostal). The folk religions of "santería and espiritismo are accepted, if not followed, by a substantial part of the [Puerto Rican] population."[23] Dominicans primarily affiliate with the Catholic church, though some Dominicans do adhere to some of the Protestant denominations. Among Dominicans, there are also some who follow and practice folk religions, such as santería and voodoo.

While there are some Protestant denominations that are popular in some areas, Roman Catholicism remains the predominant religion for most Latinos. The conservative positions of the Catholic church (i.e., abstinence until marriage, no contraceptives except for natural family planning, and the lack of openness about sexuality) have possibly contributed to the higher fertility rate among Latina women.

Religious identity, however, seems to serve as a protective factor against many risks during adolescence. Youth who feel connected to their religion and who make a vow of abstinence are more likely to delay the onset of sexual intercourse until their later adolescent years.[24] A number of studies found that adolescent females, 15-19 years of age, who felt religion was not of great significance in their lives and did not regularly attend church, were more likely to be sexually active.[25] Moreover, it does not appear that any particular denomination has any greater likelihood of predicting sexual activity.[26] The extent to which second, third, or fourth generation Latino youth embrace their religion and feel a strong religious identity is an area that needs considerably more research to determine what steps could be taken to support Latino youth's religious identity in hopes of protecting them from adolescent pregnancy and sexually transmitted diseases.

Adolescent Development

Adolescence begins with a biological event, the onset of puberty, and ends with entrance into the adult world, an unspecified event that cannot be pinpointed in time but usually coincides with commitments to marriage, work, or career. The chronological benchmarks vary, although adolescence generally begins around age 12 and is generally recognized to end at age 20. The emphasis of adolescence is on sexual development, as well as the integration of societal and family values into the identity of the individual. This stage of development facilitates the adolescent's ability to plan for the future and move away from the need for immediate gratification.

During adolescence, youth must adjust to their changing bodies, form their identities, and develop adult thinking skills. All three are directly related to teen sexuality. The dramatic biological changes that occur during the adolescent growth spurt are usually spread over a two- or three-year period. There are obvious increases in height and weight and changes in body proportion, including the appearance of sexual characteristics and the capacity to reproduce. A critical aspect of adolescents' understanding of selfhood involves coming to terms with their changing bodies. Adolescents must adapt to their own body changes in appearance and function, as well as to the responses of other persons to those changes.

The dramatic physiological changes occur in tandem with a major psychological event: the adolescent quest for personal identity. In the Latino culture, children are taught at an early age that the needs of the family are more important than the needs of the individual. This value may lead to increased stress upon Latino youth as they begin to become acculturated in the wider culture.

During adolescence, teens begin to switch from identification with their parents to increased identification with their peers. Research suggests that adolescents often seek out peers whose beliefs, values, and even behaviors are similar to those of their families. While peer and other social influences often reinforce familial values, some influences may expose the adolescent to values that differ significantly from the family's. Thus, the need to balance peer pressure and family expectations creates both new challenges and family tensions as adolescents begin to make independent decisions. These challenges are exacerbated for Latino teens who are placed in the position of accepting traditional family values *and* integrating into the wider society.

Adolescence is a time for trying out new behaviors. Although experimentation is essential for development, it may also lead to an increase in risky behaviors—and adolescents are likely to underestimate the potential for negative consequences.

Notes

1   *SIECUS Report* 25 (5), 15-16, (June-July 1997).

2   Alan Guttmacher Institute. (1994). *Sex and America's teenagers.* New York: The Alan Guttmacher Institute.

3   National Council of La Raza. (1998). *Agenda newsletter, 14* (1).

4   National Council of La Raza 1998.

5   National Council of La Raza 1998.

6   National Latina Institute for Reproductive Health. (April 1998). *Latina health: Challenges and change.* Washington, DC: Author.

7   Federal Interagency Forum on Child and Family Statistics. (1998). *America's children: Key national indicators of well-being, 1998.* Washington, DC: U.S. Government Printing Office.

8   National Center for Health Statistics. (1997). *Health, United States: 1996-97.* Hyattsville, MD: Public Health Service.

9   Federal Interagency Forum on Child and Family Statistics 1998.

10 Federal Interagency Forum on Child and Family Statistics 1998.

11 F. Mendoza. (Winter 1994). The health of Latino children in the United States. *The Future of Children, 4* (3), 43-72.

12 Mendoza 1994.

13 R. Suro. (January 25, 1999). Gore proposes school funds for Hispanics. *The Washington Post,* A10.

14 R. Rumberger. (1991). Current realities of Chicano schooling, in *Chicano school success and failure.* New York: The Falmer Press. J. Solis. (1995). The status of Latino children and youth: Challenges and prospects. In R. Zambrana (Ed.), *Understanding Latino families: Scholarship, policy, and practice.* Thousand Oaks, CA: Sage Publications. I. P. Alicea. (September 19, 1997). "No more excuses" about Hispanic dropouts. *Hispanic Outlook in Higher Education 8,* 6-7.

15 Alicea 1997.

16 Federal Interagency Forum on Child and Family Statistics 1998.

17 Suro 1999.

18 National Center for Educational Statistics data. Cited in L. Perlstein. (December 1, 1998). Tough subject: Lowering Latino dropout rate. *The Washington Post,* A3.

19 Solis 1995.

20 Perlstein 1998.

21 L. Duany & K. Pittman. (1990). *Latino youth at a crossroads.* Washington, DC: Children's Defense Fund.

22 R. W. Blum & P. M. Reinhardt. (1997). *Reducing the risk: Connections that make a difference in the lives of youth.* Minneapolis, MN: University of Minnesota, Division of General Pediatrics and Adolescent Health.

23 Committee for Hispanic Children and Families, Inc. (March 1995). *Hispanic youth at risk of pregnancy.* New York: Author.

24 Blum & Reinhardt 1997.

25 B. L. Devany & K. S. Hubley. (1981). *The determinants of adolescent pregnancy and childbearing: Final report to the National Institute of Child Health and Human Development.* Washington, DC: Mathematica Policy Research. J. K. Inazu & G. L. Fox. (1980). Maternal influence on the sexual behavior of teenage daughters. *Journal of Family Issues, 1*, 81-102. M. J. Zelnik, J. Kantner, & K. Ford. (1981). *Sex and pregnancy in adolescence.* Beverly Hills, CA: Sage Publications. S. L. Jessor & R. Jessor. (1975). Transition from virginity to nonvirginity among youth: A social-psychological study over time. *Developmental Psychology, 11* (4), 473-484. All cited in National Research Council, Panel on Adolescent Pregnancy and Childbearing. (1987). C. D. Hayes (Ed.), *Risking the future: Adolescent sexuality, pregnancy, and childbearing*, Vol. 1. Washington, DC: National Academy of Sciences.

26 National Research Council 1987.

4.Sexual Activity, Contraceptive Use, and Sexually Transmitted Diseases

Latina adolescents are twice as likely as whites to give birth, were less likely to be informed about human sexuality and birth control, and were less likely to have used contraceptives during intercourse. This chapter offers an in-depth examination of these concerns.

Sexual Activity

Recent research compares the sexual activity of African American, Latino, and white adolescents by race. For example, according to the Urban Institute, the age of onset of sexual intercourse for Latino youth falls between that of African Americans and whites: by the age of 17, 50% of Latino teens report having intercourse, compared to age 16 for African Americans and age 18 for whites.[1] The age of initiation of sexual intercourse varies for Latino adolescent males and females. Males tend to initiate sex at 13.9 years of age, two years earlier than females, at 15.9 years of age. However, significant inter-ethnic and intergroup differences exist that are not often addressed. Day[2] emphasizes that it is inaccurate to characterize *all* Latino males as being between African Americans and whites when comparing age at first intercourse. Day's research found that Mexican American men are not significantly different from white men for age of sexual debut.

The age of initiation of sexual intercourse for Latinas also varies with ethnicity. Latinas overall report an average age of 15 for initiating sexual intercourse, with Mexican American Latinas starting slightly older, at 16. Additionally, studies have looked at the impact of the acculturation process on Latinas' age of initiation of sexual intercourse and rates of sexual activity. Among Mexican American adolescent females, generational differences exist: Mexican-born adolescent females report having a later age of onset of sexual activity (between age 17-19), while U.S.-born Mexican American females report having initiated sexual intercourse between the ages of 15-17. Additionally, Mexican-born adolescent females report having fewer partners than U.S.-born adolescent females.[3]

A current study that examined the effectiveness of HIV/STD and pregnancy prevention programs for urban middle school students in Northern California found that, among different ethnicities, Latinos were most likely to report having a boyfriend or girlfriend who was older. The older the boyfriend or girlfriend, the more likely that the youth had had first intercourse by the sixth grade. The boys who were dating were more likely to report having had sexual intercourse than the boys without girlfriends. For the boys, the age difference of the partner was not found to be a significant factor. For the girls, however, the age of the boyfriend was found to be significant. Not only did girls who were dating report having had sexual intercourse significantly more than those girls without boyfriends, but also those girls with older boyfriends were significantly more likely to have had sexual intercourse than girls dating someone of the same age.

Among sexually active youth, those with an older partner were more likely to have sex more frequently, to have more partners in the last 12 months, to have used drugs or alcohol during the last sexual encounter, and to have used a condom during the last sexual encounter than students with same-age partners. Girls who had an older partner, however, were no more likely to report greater condom use than girls with a same-age partner. This is a particularly important point to address when examining the cultural impact of communication among males and females around issues of contraception and sexual decisionmaking. Gender and relationship power issues within the Latino culture may prevent Latina youth with partners of any age from negotiating sexual and contraceptive choices, placing Latina female adolescents at risk for unintended pregnancy and STDs.

The number of Latino teenagers who have had sexual intercourse falls in between African Americans and whites. Between ages 15-19, the number of Latino teenagers who report having sex is 61%, significantly lower than the percentage of African American teenagers (80%), but higher than whites (50%).[4] When activity among females is compared, Latina adolescents report the lowest percentage of sexual activity: 45% of Latina adolescents have had sex, compared to 59% of African Americans, and 48% of whites.[5]

When measuring the number of partners and frequency of sex, of those Latino adolescent males who were sexually experienced, 49% had had more than one partner in the past year, compared to 53% of African Americans and 39% of whites. Mel Hovell et al. studied the sexual activity of Latino and white teens.[6] The study found that Latinas were the least sexually experienced of all gender/race groups, meaning they had fewer partners and had sex less frequently. In addition to this finding, the Latinas were less experienced than the Latino males, while there was no significant difference between white males and females. de Anda's study supports Hovell's findings.[7] For example, she reports that in a small survey among Mexican American and white female adolescents, whites had had two to three partners, compared to one among the Mexican American teens. Again, the white teens reported a higher frequency of intercourse.

Contraceptive Use

Latina youth may be more at risk of unintended pregnancy due to religious and family beliefs against contraception and premarital sex. Efforts to study family influences on the sexual behavior of teens have provided mixed results, however.[8]

Two facts remain clear: Latina adolescents report lower levels of sexual involvement and they are less likely to use contraceptives early or at all. Family or religious values that may inhibit communication between parents and children, coupled with the lack of access to health care common among Latino youth, may pose barriers to acquiring information and contraceptives.

Research regarding contraception use suggests this as a significant area for intervention. Studies show that Latino individuals have less information available on human sexuality, pregnancy prevention, and STDs, and less access to contraceptives,[9] possibly accounting for the low level of contraceptive use among Latino teens.

One study analyzed condom use among 1,198 teenage males, ages 15 to 19, in 1988. Latino males were less likely to use condoms than African American or white teens.[10] Similarly, in a comparison of females, Latinas were less likely than either African American or white female teens to use a contraceptive.[11]

A comparison by the Urban Institute found that condom use in 1995 among Latino adolescents remained significantly less than African Americans or whites: 71% of sexually active adolescent Latino males reported using condoms *inconsistently or not at all*, compared to 54% of whites and 53% of African Americans.[12] Among Latino youth, a sizable proportion reported that they were not using any contraceptives, and for those that were, a large number reported relying almost exclusively on withdrawal. This lack of contraception use among Latino adolescents magnifies their vulnerability for unintended pregnancy.

In addition, certain characteristics of teenage sex among all teens may leave Latino adolescents particularly at risk. The Alan Guttmacher Institute suggests characteristics of teenage sex that may leave youth on the whole more vulnerable to unintended pregnancy and STDs. These may have an even more significant impact on Latino youth:

- First, teenagers tend to have sexual intercourse sporadically, which can affect efforts to prevent STDs and unintended pregnancy by making them less likely to be prepared when they do have intercourse.[13] Latino adolescents report the lowest frequency of sex, thus the most sporadic. This may contribute to the lack of planning or contraceptive use.

- Second, the necessary communication and agreement regarding contraception may be more difficult for teens whose partners are significantly older. As de Anda reported, the presence of older partners is common among Mexican American female adolescents.[14] The age of their partners was significantly older—on average five years.

Research indicates a third and more troubling characteristic of adolescent sexual intercourse that could contribute to Latina teens' lack of contraceptive use and unplanned sexual activity. Flores et al. report that Mexican American adolescent females indicated a vulnerability for engaging in unwanted sex.[15] This finding is consistent with research reporting that many Latina women, similar to white and African American women, experience some form of sexual coercion from their male partners.[16]

Sexually Transmitted Diseases (STDs)

Compared with older adults, adolescents (10- to 19-year-olds) are at higher risk for acquiring STDs for a number of reasons: they may be more likely to have multiple sexual partners rather than a single, long-term relationship; they may be more likely to engage in un-protected intercourse; and they may select partners at higher risk. During the past two decades, the age of initiation of sexual activity has steadily decreased and age at first marriage has increased, re-sulting in increases in premarital sexual experience among adoles-cent women and in an enlarging pool of young women at risk. In addition, the higher prevalence of STDs among Latino adolescents reflects multiple barriers to quality STD prevention services, includ-ing lack of insurance or other ability to pay, lack of transportation, discomfort with facilities and services designed for English-speaking adults, and concerns about confidentiality.[17]

According to the Centers for Disease Control and Prevention, every year approximately 3 million American teenagers acquire an STD. The most serious of these infections is HIV and the develop-ment of AIDS. Although Latinos comprise only 12% of the 13- to 19-year-old group, they account for 18% of the cases of AIDS reported for this age group.[18]

Latinos represent 17% of all cases of AIDS among men and 20% of the total number of cases reported among women. For Latino men, the current AIDS case rate (the number of cases relative to population size) is nearly three times that for white men (94.5 cases per 100,000, compared to 32.5 cases per 100,000). For women, the rate is six times higher (23 cases per 100,000, compared to 3.8 cases per 100,000).[19]

Notes

1   F. L. Sonenstein, K. Stewart, L. Duberstein Lingberg, M. Pernas, & S. Williams. (1997). *Involving males in teen pregnancy: A guide for program planners.* Washington, DC: The Urban Institute.

2   R. Day. (November 1992). The transition to first intercourse among racially and culturally diverse youth. *Journal of Marriage and the Family, 54,* 749-762.

3   E. Flores, S. Eyre, & S. Millstein. (1998). Sociocultural beliefs related to sex among Mexican American adolescents. *Hispanic Journal of Behavioral Health Sciences, 20* (1), 60-82.

4   Sonenstein et al. 1997.

5   Alan Guttmacher Institute. (1993). *Teenage sexual and reproductive behavior.* Facts in Brief. New York: Author.

6   M. Hovell, C. Sipan, E. Blumberg, C. Atkins, C. R. Hofstetter, & S. Kreiter. (November 1994). Family influences on Latino and Anglo adolescents sexual behavior. *Journal of Marriage and the Family, 56,* 973-986.

7   D. de Anda, R. M. Becerra, & E. Fielder. (August 1990). In their own words: The life experiences of Mexican-American and white pregnant adolescents and adolescent mothers. *Child and Adolescent Social Work, 7* (4), 301-318.

8   Hovell et al. 1994.

9   A. Marcell. (1994). Understanding ethnicity, identity formation, and risk behavior among adolescents of Mexican descent. *Journal of School Health, 64* (8).

10 F. Mendoza. (Winter 1994). The health of Latino children in the United States. *The Future of Children 4,* (3), 43-72.

11 Alan Guttmacher Institute 1994.

12 Sonenstein et al. 1997.

13 Alan Guttmacher Institute. (1994). *Sex and America's teenagers.* New York: The Alan Guttmacher Institute.

14 de Anda 1990.

15 Flores et al. 1998.

16 Flores et al. 1998.

17 Division of STD Prevention. (September 1996). Sexually transmitted disease surveillance, 1995. U.S. Department of Health and Human Services, Public Health Service. Atlanta, GA: Centers for Disease Control and Prevention.

18 Alan Guttmacher Institute 1994.

19 Kaiser Family Foundation National Survey of Latinos on HIV/AIDS. (1998). Available on-line at http://www.kff.org.

5. Marriage and Childbearing

Since 1991, teen pregnancy and birth rates have declined. After increasing sharply in the late 1980s, birth rates declined for American teenagers from 1991 through 1997.[1] Declines were reported for all race and ethnic origin groups, with the largest declines found for African American teenagers. Since 1991, the rate for Latino teenagers has declined by a total of 7.1%. Between 1996 and 1997, preliminary data revealed that birth rates for Latino teenagers fell 3%[2]; however, they continue to be substantially higher than those for other racial groups, except African American teens. This chapter presents information on rates among Latino adolescents for childbearing and marriage.

Perceptions of Marriage and Childbearing

In a study of girls enrolled in grades 6-8 at four public schools in southern California, it was reported that Latina girls want their first birth and marriage to be at an earlier age than their African American and white counterparts. Further, Latina girls reported the youngest best age of first birth (21.9 years), desired age at first birth (23.3), and desired age at marriage (22.1). Latino girls place the least importance on educational and career goals and were most pessimistic about achieving those goals. As respondents' age increased and as their educational and career aspirations decreased, they became more likely to intend to have sexual intercourse in the near future. Latino respondents were similar to Southeast Asians in being influenced by their mothers' age at marriage and first birth; furthermore, as Latina girls' family incomes rose, they became less likely to intend to have sexual intercourse soon.[3]

Finally, the study examined school and job prospects. Among all respondents except Latina girls, positive educational and job aspirations were associated with a low perceived likelihood of a nonmarital birth. Latina girls from families with low incomes were more likely to expect that they would experience a nonmarital birth than were those from wealthier families; this perception was also found among those who were born in the United States and those who had been living in the United States for many years.[4]

Marriage

Many point out that early childbearing is more culturally acceptable in the Latino community and that many teenagers who give birth are married. Indeed, Latinos are more likely to marry during adolescence; in 1997, 14% of 18- to 19-year-old Latina women were married, compared to 6% of whites and 4% of African Americans in that age group.[5] It is equally important to note, however, that the rate of those who are married has declined. Some researchers believe that, as Latinos become acculturated, the rate of marriage among Latino teenagers will decrease.

A factor in the levels of nonmarital childbearing observed for Latina women is related to the relatively high incidence of cohabitation among Latino couples. Birth certificate data provide additional evidence of this. The birth certificate used in Puerto Rico distinguishes between unmarried women who are living with the father of the child and unmarried women who are not living with the father. According to 1995 data, three-quarters of the unmarried women who gave birth were living with the father of the child.[6]

Childbearing

Latina teens are more likely to give birth when they become pregnant,[7] which contributes to the higher birthrates.[8] Latina adolescents may have adopted traditional Hispanic cultural values that make it acceptable to become an adolescent mother and have a family.[9] Although a positive, functional occurrence in an agrarian society, teenage marriage and childbearing becomes a negative one in light of the economic reality that immigrant Latino families are forced to accept in this society.

The Latino adolescent birth rate for 15- to 19-year-olds fell marginally from 101.8 births per 1,000 in 1996 to 99.1 per 1,000 in 1997.[10] Yet, even with the slight decrease, Latino teens still have the highest adolescent birthrate compared to African American teens (89.5 per 1,000 in 1997) and non-Hispanic whites (36.4 per 1,000 in 1997). Among births to all Latino women in 1997, births to Latino adolescents accounted for 17%, compared to 10% for whites and 23% for African Americans. There are significant subgroup differences in the Latino population, however. In 1996, the proportion of births to teenage mothers among Cuban women was only 8%; among Central and South American women, 11%; among Mexican and "other/ unknown" Latino women, 18-20%; with the highest proportion among Puerto Rican women, at 23%.[11] Examining the proportion of births to teenagers may be useful in gauging the impact of adolescent childbearing on a population.

There is a distinctive pattern in the levels of age-specific birth rates by race and Latino origin and the rates vary substantially.

Among teenagers 15-19 years, rates are highest for Mexican teenagers (120.7 per 1,000 in 1996) followed by African American (94.2), Puerto Rican (82.3), and American Indian teenagers (73.9 per 1,000). The rates for non-Hispanic white (37.6), Cuban (34.0), and Asian Pacific Islander (24.6) teenage subgroups are considerably lower. Among teenage subgroups 15-17 and 18-19 years, the patterns were generally similar to those for all teenagers 15-19 years. Rates were highest for Mexican teenagers and lowest for Asian Pacific Islander teenagers. These relationships were observed in each year, 1994-1996. Prior to 1994, birth rates had been highest for African American teenagers. (See Figures 3 and 4.)

Between 1995 and 1996, teenage birth rates declined for all groups except Cuban teenagers, for whom the rate increased from 29.2 to 34.0 per 1,000. The declines were 3% and 4%, respectively, for Mexican and white teenagers. Other declines were 5% for African American teenagers, 8% for Puerto Rican, and 10% for other Latino teenagers. From 1991, when rates for teenagers generally were at a peak, to 1996, birth rates fell 20 to 21% for African American, Puerto Rican, and other Latino teens. Declines for white teens were less, at 13%.[12]

Prenatal care utilization, which provides opportunities for professional medical advice and detection and management of preexisting medical conditions, can promote healthier pregnancy outcomes. The proportion of Latino teens who began prenatal care in the first trimester improved. For Latina teens under 15 years of age, 50% began prenatal care in the first trimester and for 15- to 19-year-olds, 63% began in first trimester. A decrease was noted in the percent of Latina teens who had late or no prenatal care: 15% of under 15-year-olds and 9.2% of 15- to 19-year-olds had late or no care. By comparison, among African American teen mothers 15 to 19 years of age, 9% had late or no care, versus 5% for white teen mothers 15 to 19 years of age. (See Figure 5.)

Figure 3. Birth Rate for Females Ages 15 to 17 by Race and Latino Origin, 1980-97

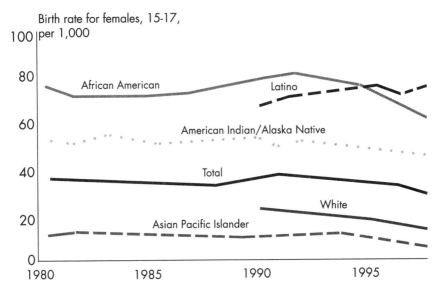

Note: Rates from 1981–1989 were not calculated for Hispanics or non-Hispanic whites, because estimates for populations were not available. 1997 data are preliminary.

Tobacco use during pregnancy is associated with a variety of adverse outcomes, including low birthweight, intrauterine growth retardation, and infant mortality, as well as negative consequences for child health and development. Maternal smoking among teenagers increased about 2% overall, but among young teenagers aged 15 to 17 years, the rate rose 5% to 15.4%, with an even greater relative increase for African American teenagers, from 4.3 to 5%. Smoking rates rose as well in 1996 for Mexican and Puerto Rican teenagers aged 15 to 17 years. Despite these increases, smoking rates for non-Hispanic white teenagers are still four to six times the rates for Latino teenagers.

Figure 4. Percent of Teen Births That Occurred to Unmarried Teens by Race/Ethnicity, 1996

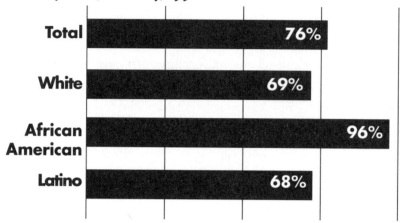

Source: The Annie B. Casey Foundation, from data compiled by the National Center for Health Statistics. (1998). *When teens have sex: Issues and trends.* Kids Count Special Report.

Figure 5. Percent of Births to Teens Receiving Inadequate Prenatal Care by Race/Ethnicity, 1996

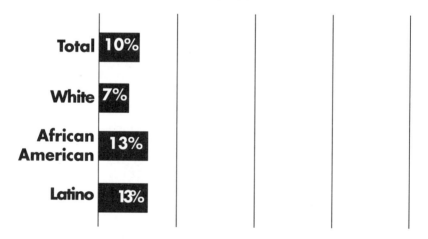

Source: The Annie B. Casey Foundation, from data compiled by the National Center for Health Statistics. (1998). *When teens have sex: Issues and trends. Kids Count Special Report.*

Another important measure for the Latino population is the proportion of births to adolescents born in the United States, as compared to foreign-born Latino adolescents. Here the differences are very substantial, with twice as many teenage mothers among U.S.-born Latino adolescents as among foreign-born Latina adolescents (26.1% compared to 12.0%, respectively). Again, considerable differences exist among the subgroups. For Mexican teens, the percent of teenage mothers among U.S.-born adolescents is 27.2%, compared to 12.5% for foreign born; for Puerto Rican adolescents it is 25.3%, compared to 19.8%; for Cuban adolescents, 12.1% compared to 5.0%; for Central and South American adolescents, 23.5% compared to 9.6; and for adolescents of "other and unknown Latino" origin, the proportion of teenage mothers among U.S.-born Latino adolescents is 23.2% compared to 10.1%.[13] These last figures highlight the impact of the acculturation process for Latino adolescents in the United States.

Notes

1   S. J. Ventura, R. N. Anderson, J. A. Martin, & B. L. Smith. (1998). *Births and deaths: Preliminary data for 1997. National vital statistics report, Vol. 47, No. 4.* Hyattsville, MD: National Center for Health Statistics.

2   Ventura et al. 1998.

3   Alan Guttmacher Institute. (September/October 1998). Expectations about marriage and childbearing vary by race and ethnicity among girls in grades 6-8. *Family Planning Perspectives, 30* (5), 252-253.

4   *Family Planning Perspectives, 30* (5), 252-253.

5 T. A. Lugeia. (1998). Marital status and living arrangements, March 1997 (Update). Current Population Reports P-20, No. 506. Washington, DC: U.S. Bureau of the Census.

6 T. J. Mathews, S. J. Ventura, S. C. Curtin, & J. A. Martin. (1998). *Births of Hispanic origin, 1989-95.* Monthly vital statistics report, Vol. 46, No. 6, Supplement. Hyattsville, MD: National Center for Health Statistics.

7 A. Marcell. (1994). Understanding ethnicity, identity formation, and risk behavior among adolescents of Mexican descent. *Journal of School Health, 64* (8).

8 D. de Anda, R. M. Becerra, & E. Fielder. (August 1990). In their own words: The life experiences of Mexican-American and white pregnant adolescents and adolescent mothers. *Child and Adolescent Social Work, 7* (4), 301-318. A. Marcell. (1994). Understanding ethnicity, identity formation, and risk behavior among adolescents of Mexican descent. *Journal of School Health, 64* (8).

9 C. Brindis. (1992). Adolescent pregnancy prevention for Hispanic youth. *Journal of School Health, 62* (7).

10 S. J. Ventura, J. A. Martin, S. C. Curtin, & T. J. Mathews. (1998). *Report of final natility statistics, 1996.* Monthly vital statistics report, Vol. 46, No. 11, Supplement. Hyattsville, MD: National Center for Health Statistics.

11 Ventura et al. 1998.

12 Ventura et al. 1998.

13 Ventura et al. 1998.

6. Approaches to Adolescent Pregnancy Prevention

Adolescent pregnancy prevention programs vary widely in program model and intervention techniques. There has been little rigorous evaluation of the prevention programs already in place, however, and even less evaluation of program models aimed at intervening in the Latino community. Similarly, an adolescent pregnancy prevention program that may have been implemented successfully in a Mexican American community may not work when replicated in a Cuban community or other ethnic groups in the Latino community.

A number of factors have been identified in the adolescent pregnancy prevention research as antecedents to early adolescent sexual activity and pregnancy. Prevention programs aimed at Latino communities should try to incorporate not only identified risk factors and what is known to work from the research in adolescent pregnancy prevention, but also incorporate the context of the cultural norms and expectations of the Latino community and the larger community with which the youth interact.

According to research done at Child Trends, Inc.,[1] prevention programs must do more than simply address youth's attitudes, beliefs, knowledge, and skills to bring about changes in sexual behavior. Prevention programs should strive to enhance family relationships and build upon the assets of adolescents, as well as address some of the main antecedents of adolescent pregnancy, such as poverty, disadvantages, school failure, and poor academic performance.

Though not much research has been done to directly link the "best bets" for what works in adolescent pregnancy prevention efforts to Latino adolescent pregnancy prevention programs, several program approaches exist that may hold promise for replication within Latino communities.

Health Education

Sexuality education programs come in two basic varieties: abstinence-only education and comprehensive sexuality education. Abstinence-only education programs focus on abstaining from sexual intercourse, with some promoting abstaining from sexual intercourse until marriage. Abstinence-only programs often promote abstinence as the *only* way to avoid the risk of pregnancy and STDs. They usually omit information about contraception or discuss contraception only in the context of its failure to protect against pregnancy and STDs. Of the relatively little research done on abstinence-only education programs, studies are often cited as showing that the abstinence-only programs reviewed had no effect on delaying the age of first intercourse.[2]

Comprehensive sexuality education programs often have an abstinence-based approach, providing youth with age-, gender-, and culture-appropriate information on the use of abstinence and contraception as methods of protection against STDs and early, unintended pregnancy. The goals of comprehensive sexuality education are

- to give youth accurate information on human sexuality;

- to allow youth to explore their own attitudes, beliefs, and values regarding sexuality;
- to provide the opportunity for youth to learn and practice skills for successful relationships; and
- to enhance youth's ability to productively take responsibility for issues of abstinence, sexual pressures, and negotiating contraception in the context of a healthy relationship.[3]

Those comprehensive sexuality programs that provide a clear message and information—combined with activities for youth to discuss the impact of media messages and peer pressures and activities to practice communication, negotiation, and behavior modeling—have been found to increase the age of sexual initiation slightly and moderately increase the use of contraceptives as well.[4] A common concern among many communities is that discussing sexual intercourse and contraceptive methods will encourage youth to become sexually active. Studies have shown that providing comprehensive sexuality education to youth does not lead to an earlier age of sexual initiation.[5]

Comprehensive sexuality education programs are not necessarily always based in an educational setting. Some may take the form of after-school programs or programs run through community centers. These latter locations may have a greater chance of reaching those youth who are disconnected from the educational system.

Sexuality Education for Parents & Children

Research on parent-child communication presents a complex dynamic with varying effectiveness in preventing early initiation of sexual intercourse, depending on the presence, context, and content of the parent-child discussions. Few of the studies have involved a significantly large enough Latino population to be able to come to any conclusions about parent-child communication in Latino households.

A study of parent-child communication among Mexican and Central American youth found that "Latina adolescents who were not pregnant reported receiving more information from their parents about sexuality."[6] Another study[7] found that there was a relationship between parent-child communication about delaying sexual intercourse and less sexually active adolescents only when the parents disapproved of adolescents engaging in sexual intercourse.

Additionally, studies have found that birth control was the topic least likely to be addressed among parents and daughters: "Forty-five percent of the pregnant and parenting adolescents and 39% of the never-pregnant adolescents reported never receiving information from their parents on this topic."[8] Parental discomfort with the topic of birth control is often cited, not only among Latino parents, but among African American and white parents as well, as a major reason for avoiding the discussion.

Another striking fact that has implications for prevention programs is that the pregnant or parenting Latina adolescents in the Flores study were more likely to come from families that were not intact: "The strong relationship between non-intact families and adolescent pregnancy suggests that intervention involving parents should allow for the inclusion of other significant resource adults since the parents may often be unavailable in the highest risk families."[9]

Many experts agree that community and family involvement in broad-based approaches are an essential component to protecting youth from premature parenthood and STDs. The Plain Talk Initiative, supported by the Annie E. Casey Foundation, works with neighborhoods to facilitate communication about sexuality among adults and youth. The Plain Talk Initiative has been implemented in a number of communities, including Barrio Logan (or Logan Heights) in San Diego, California. The participants of Plain Talk found that, while certain components of the program could be replicated across communities, "They also discovered ... that each community's approach needed to be tailored to the unique personality and history of its residents."[10]

The Barrio Logan community is made up primarily of people of Mexican heritage and Spanish is the dominant language spoken in homes and on the streets.

> Hablando Claro [Plain Talk] strives to work within the cultural richness of its people. "We have many strong customs and traditions that help to keep us a strong people," explained Marta Flores [Director of Hablando Claro]. "But at the same time, we have a cultural silence that hurts us. And now in the light of HIV / AIDS it's more than just an issue of having a baby."[11]

Using community mapping and assessment, coupled with the active participation of the residents, adults and adolescents, teachers, neighbors, health service providers, church leaders, and many more, Plain Talk staff created a curriculum that was "culturally and linguistically appropriate, and at the same time encouraged adults to rethink how they viewed issues of sex and sexuality and to consider discussing these issues with youth."[12]

Contraceptive Services

Contraceptive access programs include family planning services, school-based health centers, and school condom availability programs. There is speculation that family planning services which provide other services outside of the strictly medical problems (e.g, psychosocial services, information, and counseling) are more likely to be used by adolescents. In addition, improvements to clinic protocol that include trying to involve the adolescent's parents or partners more, and postponing the physical examination until the second visit have been suggested to increase the likelihood of adolescents attending a clinic.[13]

School-based health centers and condom availability programs provide an opportunity for youth to access free, confidential health care and contraceptives within the context of their own school. This is a beneficial situation to the many Latino students who are underinsured or lack access to health care in the community. One of the downsides to this type of prevention effort is that it misses a segment of the youth population that are at high risk for early pregnancy and STDs—those youth that have already dropped out of the school system and/or have been placed in residential facilities.[14]

Some communities voice concerns about the availability of condoms in the schools influencing youth to either become sexually active or become more sexually active. There is no research providing evidence to support this claim. Students who use condoms simply obtain them from the school rather than going elsewhere. There is an equal lack of strong evidence to support the theory that condom availability programs increase actual condom use among already sexually active youth.[15]

Male Responsibility

There has been a recent movement toward including adolescent males in teenage pregnancy prevention work. Historically, efforts have focused mainly on females, omitting an important piece of the adolescent pregnancy problem: males. More research has recently become available on how to best reach the teenage male population. This has come in part from The National Survey of Adolescent Males, begun in 1988, which seeks to identify trends in young males' behavior and attitudes.[16] In addition, promising work is taking place in the field, which involves Latino males in prevention.

Male involvement programs have begun to focus on a number of factors that have become both political and social concerns lately: specifically, STD prevention, child support, statutory rape laws, and fatherhood. There has been an added emphasis on reaching males in their early twenties, since research shows that many older teenage females (age 17, 18, and 19) have male partners who are in their twenties.[17] This male age group is typically not targeted in pregnancy prevention efforts. In the Latino community, where it may be more culturally acceptable for a younger female to have an older male partner, programs that address cultural differences and cultural stereotypes, provide education on child support and statutory rape laws, and facilitate young men taking an active, responsible role in pregnancy prevention and in fatherhood, may be especially beneficial to young Latino males.

Adolescent males can be reached in a variety of social settings, the most likely being through school, work, health care, or sports. In addition, approximately half of adolescent males who have not yet had sexual intercourse often are involved in youth groups or clubs. A disturbing statistic that cannot be ignored is that "three quarters of the teenage males with past criminal involvement, including ever being picked up by the police, arrested, or jailed, are also sexually experienced."[18] Half of sexually experienced males and 22% of males who are still virgins are involved in the criminal justice system. Developing male involvement programs to reach teenage males through the criminal justice system may be an untraditional—and yet important—intervention strategy. There are also a large number of adolescent males in the nation's child welfare system, either in foster care, residential treatment, or independent living, who go largely unreached by any pregnancy prevention efforts.

Hombres Jovenes con Palabra is a program for young men to increase awareness and responsibility of pregnancy prevention among other young men. The program was developed in 1988 by Jerry Tello in response to a lack of culturally competent programs for adolescent males. The comprehensive program seeks to engage males and emphasize the importance of responsibility, using the "indigenous Latino concept of *El Hombre Noble* (the noble man) as the foundation of male responsibility."[19] The curriculum centers around the notion of being a man of *palabra* (word) and the principle that a man of word "follows through with what he says he will do."[20]

The program builds upon the strengths of Latino culture to help young Latino males address their conceptions of manhood, machismo, and maleness. Sessions explore sexual responsibility, the consequences of risk-taking, and the deeper underpinnings of unintended adolescent pregnancy, including gender and racial stereotypes, family functioning, and societal expectations.[21] The Hombres Jovenes program has been successfully adapted to reach at-risk youth in schools and correctional facilities, as well as mainstream classroom settings and youth leadership groups.

Youth Development

"The problem in many of the Latino communities," says Aracely Panameno of the Latina Reproductive Health Institute, "is a lack of hope for the future." Early childbearing among any population "appears to be strongly related to limited life options."[22] The main goal in Positive Youth Development is to improve life options for youth by involving them in their community and building on assets.

Search Institute has named 40 developmental assets that youth need to grow into healthy, capable, and caring adults. These assets fall into two categories: external (support, empowerment, boundaries, expectations, and constructive use of time), and internal (commitment to learning, positive values, social competencies, and positive identity).[23]

The asset-building approach to youth development is not a program model, nor a "how-to" outline. It is a philosophy that places the developmental needs of young people at the foundation of every effective prevention effort. Youth development programs allow young people to be not only competent, but connected, caring, and committed. In addition to skills, young people must have a solid sense of safety and structure, membership and belonging, mastery and purpose, responsibility, and self-worth. Youth development programs provide young people with opportunities to which they can say yes.

In 1995, Oklahoma City was one of the 13 communities selected by the Centers for Disease Control and Prevention as a part of a community-based teen pregnancy prevention initiative, called the

"Heart of OKC—Healthy, Empowered And Responsible Teens of OKC." For OKC, assets have been defined as "attitudes, knowledge, values, skills, and relationships that strengthen the ability of individuals to become healthy, capable, responsible adults." The nine key assets for OKC are aspirations for the future; constructive use of time; cultural respect (sensitivity to cultural issues); skills for meaningful employment; decisionmaking, especially related to refusal skills, restraint, and personal health; positive family communication; positive peer role models; relationships with non-parent adults; and service to others.

Examples of Heart of OKC interventions that link teen pregnancy prevention and health promotion with youth development include the following:

- "Learn and Serve" community service projects funded through the State Department of Education;

- Skill-building projects partnered with local business, such as Home Depot;

- A Junior League project that assists homeless youth in completing high school; and

- A replication of the "Postponing Sexual Involvement" (PSI) curriculum that uses high school teens as program leaders.

Multicomponent Programs

Multicomponent programs use a variety (two or more) of approaches at one time to decrease rates of teen pregnancy. Programs may involve sexuality education through the schools, media campaigns, family planning and condom availability services, schoolwide activities, and the active participation of churches and other community organizations. Because of the multifaceted approach, evaluation efforts have been difficult. There is some evidence to support the theory that the more intensive and long-term the programs are, the greater the impact on adolescent sexual behavior.[24]

Michael Carrera calls The Children's Aid Society's model a "long term, holistic, multidimensional adolescent sexuality and pregnancy...program for young people, parents, and adults."[25] This model, which was developed in Harlem in a predominantly African American and Latino community, is far from the traditional educational approach to pregnancy prevention. Working on the theory that adolescent pregnancy is a symptom of much larger problems of hopelessness and limited life options, the program implements a variety of methods of reaching youth and empowering them to achieve a meaningful life as well as reduce the incidence of teenage pregnancy, substance abuse, and violence. Many young people in the program live daily in conditions of disruptive home situations, poverty, racism, and limited access to decent employment and educational opportunities. In the face of such desperate circumstances, it is little wonder some adolescents do not see teenage pregnancy or premature parenting as a negative outcome.

The program's seven main areas include the Job Club and Career Awareness Component, the Family Life and Sex Education Component, Medical and Health Services, Mental Health Services, the Academic Assessment and Homework Help Component, Self-Esteem Through the Performing Arts, and the Lifetime Sports Component.

Implications for Latino Adolescent Pregnancy Prevention

While many of these approaches to adolescent pregnancy prevention have been implemented among white and African American teenagers, there has been very little replication of programs for Latino adolescents. Major issues that should be addressed when working with Latino adolescents are cultural and religious values closely linked to birth, marriage, and contraception; low educational attainment and school progress; limited education and occupational plans; and higher rate of intended teen fertility compared with whites and African American. Programs should be developed that address multiple factors, including family and cultural concepts of marriage, sexuality and fertility (intergenerational differences, gender roles, and inequality in interpersonal relationships); educational and career options for males and females; and access to reproductive health services.[26]

Notes

1   K. A. Moore, B. W. Sugland, C. Blumenthal, D. Glei, & N. Snyder (June 1995). *Adolescent pregnancy prevention programs: Interventions and evaluations.* Washington, DC: Child Trends, Inc.

2   W. Castro. (1998). *Welfare reform and abstinence education.* Washington, DC: CWLA Press.

3   National Guidelines Task Force. (1992). *Guidelines for comprehensive sexuality education, kindergarten - 12th grade.* New York: SIECUS.

4   Moore et al. 1995

5   Moore et al. 1995.

6   L. M. Baumeister, E. Flores, & B. V. Marin. (1995). Sex information given to Latina adolescents by parents." *Health Education Research: Theory and Practice, 10*(2), 233-239.

7   J. Jaccard & P. Dittus. (1991). Parent-teen communication: Toward the prevention of unintended pregnancies. New York: Springer-Verlag. Cited in Baumeister et al. 1995.

8   Baumeister et al. 1995.

9   Baumeister et al. 1995.

10 The Annie E. Casey Foundation. (1998). *Plain talk: The storyof a community-based strategy to reduce teen pregnancy.* Baltimore, MD: Author.

11 The Annie E. Casey Foundation 1998.

12 The Annie E. Casey Foundation 1998.

13 B. W. Sugland. Teen pregnancy prevention: Promising approaches for Latino youth. Presented at Latino Adolescent Pregnancy Prevention Symposium, Child Welfare League of America, in Washington, D.C., November 13, 1998. D. Kirby. (1997). *No easy answers: Research findings on programs to reduce teen pregnancy.* Summary. Washington, DC: The National Campaign to Prevent Teen Pregnancy.

14 Kirby 1997.

15 Kirby 1997.

16 F. L. Sonenstein, K. Stewart, L. Duberstein Lingberg, M. Pernas, & S. Williams. (1997). *Involving males in teen pregnancy: A guide for program planners.* Washington, DC: The Urban Institute.

17 Sonenstein et al. 1997.

18 Sonenstein et al. 1997.

19 Sonenstein et al. 1997.

20 Sonenstein et al. 1997.

21 Sonenstein et al. 1997.

22 C. Brindis. (1992). Adolescent pregnancy prevention for Hispanic youth. *Journal of School Health, 62* (7).

23 The material in this section was taken from S. Rodine. (December 1998). Teen pregnancy and prevention: A new approach. *Pregnancy Prevention for Youth: An Interdisciplinary Newsletter, 1* (2).

24 Kirby 1997.

25 M. A. Carrera. (August/September 1995). Preventing adolescent pregnancy: In hot pursuit. *SIECUS Report, 23* (6), 16-19.

26 Sugland 1998.

7.

Policy Issues

For public policy to be effective, it needs to be proactive, theoretically informed, and research-based. Recent government policy concerning adolescent pregnancy prevention has been dominated by punitive strategies to address welfare reform. While welfare reform will continue to guide the social policy agenda, there is a growing sentiment that the search for better policy results will depend on research that includes the participation of Latino researchers, program developers, and policymakers for new strategies. In this chapter, we briefly explore some key features of social policy and research within the context of reproductive health and its intersection with the Latino culture. The issues of statutory rape, abstinence education, and the right to consent to contraceptive services remain at the forefront of our nation's reproductive health agenda; however, we have paid scant attention to how these issues relate to the needs of Latino adolescents.

Statutory Rape

The Issue

Recent studies indicate that at least half of all babies born to minor women are fathered by adult men.[1] Approximately half of the recipients of welfare had their first child as a teenager and are likely to receive pubic assistance for long periods of time, at great cost to the public. These facts have prompted Congress to enact legislation to reduce adolescent childbearing and welfare costs by vigorous enforcement of statutory rape laws prohibiting sexual intercourse between adults and minors. (Statutory rape is a criminal offense generally defined as intercourse with someone who is younger than the age of consent.)[2]

The welfare reform law contained provisions to require that

> ... the U.S. Attorney General shall establish and implement a program that: studies the linkage between statutory rape and teenage pregnancy, particularly by predatory older men committing repeat offenses; and educates state and local criminal law enforcement officials on the prevention and prosecution of statutory rape ... by predatory older men ... and any link to teenage pregnancy.[3]

Following the lead of Congress, several states have reviewed their statutory rape laws and have called for more vigorous enforcement of the laws. Recently, California allocated several million dollars to support the prosecution of statutory rape cases and the provision of civil penalties.

The Facts

- Seventy-four percent of women who had intercourse before age 14 and 60% of those who had sex before age 15 report having had a forced sexual experience.[4]

- Older males, when defined as at least five years older than 15- to 17-year-old mothers, are responsible for 21% of births to unmarried women younger than 18.[5]

- According to a recent study, the age of consent in 28 states was 16 years; in most of the remaining states it was 17 or 18 years, although in one state it was 15 years and in another, 14 years. [6]

- A recent study of district attorneys in Kansas reported that they do not believe that aggressive enforcement of statutory rape laws will reduce adolescent pregnancy rates. That study is consistent with results from earlier qualitative studies, including a recent American Bar Association study that interviewed prosecutors from 48 of the largest U.S. cities.[7]

Discussion

While many in the law enforcement field see no harm in implementing a strategy of increased prosecution of statutory rape cases as a deterrent to adolescent childbearing, human services professionals question the effectiveness of such a strategy. Some providers are concerned that heightened publicity and enforcement of the law will discourage sexually active and pregnant adolescents from seeking medical care for fear of having to disclose information on their partners.[8] Disclosure of information to authorities may also jeopardize any financial support they receive.

Some providers also point to complex physical, familial, and cultural factors that determine who will marry and when, who will begin sexual activity before marriage, who will begin childbearing during adolescence, and who will bear children outside marriage. In Latin America, approximately one-half to two-thirds of young women become sexually active during their teenage years. Additionally, in Latin America and the Caribbean, 12 to 28% of women first give birth at ages 15-17.[9] It has been speculated that in Latin American cultures, men typically marry much younger women, and perhaps there is a social acceptance of this custom that transcends to the Latino population in the United States. Statistics appear to support that speculation. The 1988 National Maternal and Infant Health Survey reported that 33.8% of Latino teenage mothers had partners who were at least five years older, as compared to 26.1% for African American teenage mothers and 25.2 % for white teenage mothers.[10]

Statistics from the United Nations indicate that the average age of marriage in Latin American countries is lower than in the United States. In Mexico in 1993, 36% of brides were under age 20, as compared to only 16.5% of Mexican grooms under 20. [11] These statistics indicate that many Mexican women marry before age 20, but also that most of these teenage girls are marrying men who are over 20.

Some providers have suggested that in some cultures, the family accepts and encourages young women to have relationships with older men. Older men are more likely to provide financial support to the entire family. Latino parents, like many other parents, need assistance to effectively educate young people about sexuality and communicating about sexuality and reproductive health within the context of family values.

It is recognized that decisions about whether to file charges, to engage in plea bargaining, or to reduce or dismiss charges are at the discretion of the prosecutor. According to a 1997 American Bar Association study, "Prosecutors have enormous discretion in deciding whether or not to accept a statutory rape case for prosecution for statutory rape."[12] We are concerned that there is the potential for discriminatory prosecution of a group of people. For the U.S. Latino community, where approximately one-third of the population are immigrants, prosecution may lead to imprisonment, fines, disqualification from becoming a U.S. citizen, disfranchisement, and deportation. None of those actions will lead to a decrease in adolescent childbearing or effective family policy.

Recommendations

Concerns about older males and adolescent childbearing are warranted and have encouraged much needed debate at the statehouses; there is, however, little evidence that this type of legislation will change sexual and reproductive behaviors. Based upon the work from the Latino Adolescent Pregnancy Prevention Symposium, the Child Welfare League of America and the National Council of Latino Executives recommend the following:

1. The President should direct the Attorney General to study the impact of the statutory rape laws on the Latino community. Such a study may include the number of Latinos who are prosecuted under these laws and the number of Latinos who are deported and/or denied citizenship. The information will be included in the Attorney General's report to Congress. Such information may include the number of arrests, convictions, deportations, fines, etc. This will require the creation of systems for data collection to monitor the incidents and prevalence and to report information to policymakers and the public.

2. Raise awareness in the Latino community about U.S. statutory rape laws and how they apply to people who live here. Target stakeholders (parents, policymakers, other national organizations, and youth) and provide them with information about the current laws.

3. Adolescent pregnancy prevention programs must be broadened beyond sexuality education, contraceptive access, and improved life options to include date rape, gender equality, and self-worth. Youth should be provided with opportunities to participate in programs that promote sexual equality and employment opportunities.

4. Criminal justice and human service professionals should receive training to create awareness of cultural practices in the Latino community. Human services professionals should be able to make assessments in a culturally competent manner.

Abstinence-Only Education

The Issue

In August of 1996, President Clinton signed into law the Personal Responsibility and Work Reconciliation Act of 1996. One provision in this welfare reform legislation mandated that $50 million be provided per year to the states through a Maternal and Child Health Block Grant to fund "abstinence-only until marriage" education programs. In addition to education, a state has the option to use the funds to undertake "where appropriate, mentoring, counseling and adult supervision to promote abstinence from sexual activity, with a focus on those groups which are most likely to bear children out-of-wedlock."[13]

The provisions in the federal law define abstinence education as an educational or motivational program that "has as its exclusive purpose, teaching the social, psychological, and health gains to be realized by abstaining from sexual activity"; that "teaches abstinence from sexual activity outside of marriage as the expected standard for all school age children"; and that "teaches the importance of attaining self-sufficiency before engaging in sexual activity."[14] While there is no documented evidence that such strict programs reduce teen pregnancy or delay the age of first intercourse, proponents of this type of education used the introduction of federal funding as a government "stamp of approval" and stepped up their efforts to bring abstinence-only education to schools.[15]

The Facts

- Seventeen percent of youth in the seventh and eighth grades reported having had sexual intercourse. For teens in high school (grades 9-12) , the percentage reporting ever having had intercourse almost triples to 49.3%.[16] More than two-thirds (66.7%) of teens reported having had sex by their senior year of high school.[17]

- The average age of sexual initiation among Latinas is 15.3 years, with Mexican Americans starting slightly older at 16 years.[18]

- Adolescent males report having first intercourse on the average of one year earlier than adolescent females. The median age at which 50% of teenage males report having had first intercourse is 16.6 years of age; for teenage females, 17.4 years of age.[19] One study found that 31% of Latino males initiated sex before age 13, versus 55% for African American and 12.5% for white males.[20]

- Relatively little research has been conducted on the effectiveness of abstinence education programs. Only six evaluative studies of abstinence-only programs have been published, and the results from these initial studies were not promising. These studies are often cited as showing that the abstinence-only programs reviewed had no effect on delaying the age of first intercourse.[21]

- Forty-nine states applied and received abstinence education funds from the Maternal and Child Health Bureau. Most states developed plans to target youth between the ages of 9 and 14, and several states have enacted legislation that mirrors the federal legislation.[22]

- An important component of sexuality education is parental/child communication; however, there is some evidence that Latino parents communicate less with their children about sexuality, and children report less sex information from parents than white youths.[23] Latinos are less likely to discuss AIDS with their children than non-Latinos.[24] Among Latino subgroups, it was reported that Mexican and Central American female adolescents were less likely to report discussing sex with their parents than other Latina adolescents.[25]

Discussion

With the infusion of abstinence-only-until-marriage funds from the federal government, many states are retreating from implementing comprehensive sexually education programs. Information found in comprehensive sexuality programs provides teens with facts on sexual development, reproductive health, interpersonal relationships, affection, intimacy, body image, and gender roles.[26] Comprehensive sexuality education programs not only cover biological facts, but also provide young people with practical information and skills regarding dating, sexual relationships, and contraceptive use.

Sexuality education programs have been shown to be successful at helping young people postpone intercourse, use contraception, and prevent STDs. Research shows that effective programs

- provide modeling and practice in communication and negotiation skills;

- reinforce clear and appropriate values to strengthen individual values and group norms against unprotected sexual activity;

- focus on reducing sexual risk-taking behaviors and use social learning theories (that focus on recognizing social influence, bolstering health-positive values, changing group norms and building social skills);

- employ active learning methods of instruction to provide students with the information they need to assess risks and avoid unprotected intercourse; and

- include activities that address social and media influence on sexual behavior.

An international study of sexuality education programs found that the best outcomes were obtained when education was given prior to the onset of sexual activity and when information about abstinence, contraception, and STD prevention were given. The same study also found that sexuality education does not encourage sexual experimentation or increased activity.[27]

In many Latino cultures, parents and family members are influential sources of knowledge, beliefs, attitudes, and values for children and youth. Many parents, however, are uncomfortable talking about sexuality issues. Many lack basic information on anatomy, express concern about the accuracy of the information, and may feel that discussing sexuality issues will cause teens to become sexually active. Some of the most effective teen sexuality education programs recognize the important role that parents play as sexuality educators of their children. These programs, such as Plain Talk, provide parents with cognitive information on sex, sexuality, and reproductive health; with communication skills to respond to young people questions and concerns; with support to examine their own fears and values; and with informational materials and support to offer encouragement to discuss sexuality issues with their children.[28]

Recommendations

To enable adolescents to make responsible choices concerning human sexuality and to minimize the risk of unintended pregnancy and sexually transmitted diseases, including AIDS, the Child Welfare League of America and the National Council of Latino Executives recommend the following:

1. The Department of Health and Human Services should evaluate the effectiveness of abstinence-only-until-marriage education in the Latino community. The findings should be reported to the Congress in the Secretary's annual report, *A National Strategy to Prevent Teen Pregnancy.*

2. DHHS and the states should provide funding for programs that promote sexuality education in the Latino community. Such programs should include adult education components, which should increase adults' comfort with the topic of sexuality, help them discuss sexuality and family planning methods with their children, and include significant community resources, since parents may often be unavailable or need support in obtaining information and skills. Special emphasis should be placed on methods to help parents discuss birth control.[29] Efforts should be made to enlist adults as peer educators to create formal and informal education opportunities to give messages that will empower residents. Programs should integrate components of the Latino culture into their services.

3. DHHS and the states should conduct additional studies on parental and familial attitudes and beliefs about teen sexuality and prevention approaches in the Latino community. Intervention should be community- and culturally based and involve strategies that focus on groups of youth, neighborhoods, and families, rather than on individual behavior. Youth and parents should be involved in identifying the

sociocultural issues that have an impact on adolescent sexuality and in designing the programs to reduce risky sexual behavior.[30]

4. DHHS and the states should conduct studies on sexual attitudes and behaviors in preadolescent Latinos, beginning in fifth grade and into middle school.

5. Conduct studies on the effects of intergenerational conflict, interparental conflict, changing gender roles, family functioning on adolescent health risk behaviors, and impact of acculturation on Latino communities.

Title X and Teenager's Right to Consent

The Issue

Title X of the Public Health Service Act, the federal family planning program, was enacted by Congress and signed into law by President Nixon in 1970. The program provides federal funds for project grants to public and private nonprofit organizations for the provision of family planning information and services—services that improve maternal and infant health, lower the incidence of unintended pregnancy, reduce the incidence of abortion, and lower rates of sexually transmitted diseases (STDs).[31]

From its inception, Title X has required that services be made available without regard to age or marital status. Title X-supported clinics have always provided confidential services to those who request them. This philosophy was challenged in 1996, when Rep. Ernest Istook (R-OK) offered an amendment that would have required family planning providers to obtain written parental consent for most minors seeking services at Title X funded clinics. A substitute amendment was passed that required Title X grantees to certify to the DHHS

Secretary that they encourage family participation. While the restrictive language was not included, it is expected that parental consent restrictions will be an issue in the 106th Congress.

The Facts

- According to 1994 data, an estimated 6.6 million women receive contraceptive services annually through the network of publicly subsidized family planning providers. Overall, 30% of these clients are younger than 20, 50% are aged 20 to 29, and 20% are aged 30 or older. A majority of the clients are whites (61%), while 19% are African American, 14% are Latinos, and 7% are Asians or some other race.[32]

- Services supported by Title X include contraceptive information and the provision of all contraceptive services, as well as gynecological examinations, basic lab tests, and other screening services for STDs and HIV, high blood pressure, anemia, and breast and cervical cancer.[33]

- Each year, publicly funded contraceptive services help women avoid 1.3 million unintended pregnancies, which would result in 534,000 births, 632,000 abortions, and 165,000 miscarriages. For every public dollar spent to provide family planning services, the public saves an average of $3 in Medicaid costs for pregnancy-related and newborn care.[34]

- Without publicly funded family planning services, an additional 386,000 teenagers would become pregnant each year. Of these, 155,000 would give birth, increasing the number of teenage births by one quarter. Just under 50,000 of these pregnancies would end in miscarriage, and 183,000 teenagers would have abortions, increasing abortions to teenagers by 58%.[35]

Discussion

During the past several years, Title X legislation has been under attack by conservative members of Congress. Efforts to eliminate the Title X program, restrict access by teenagers, and the lack of adequate funding have worked to undermine the program. In September 1997, the U.S. House of Representatives narrowly rejected a mandatory parental involvement amendment. Under the proposal, clinics receiving Title X funds had to notify a parent at least five days prior to providing contraceptive drugs or devices to a minor— unless the minor already had a parent's written consent or permission from a court to obtain a contraceptive without her parents' knowledge. By a small margin, the House acted instead to endorse current Title X policy that *encourages* but does not *require* parental involvement.

Although efforts have failed at the federal level, several state legislatures have debated the issue. In the State of Texas' 1997 budget, the legislature included a prohibition on the use of state family planning funds to provide prescription drugs, such as birth control pills and medication for treating sexually transmitted diseases, to minors without parental consent. The measure was invalidated by a state court, because it conflicted with the federal Title X program that supports confidential family planning services for minors. At the Governor's request, however, the state attorney general is appealing the ruling.[36]

Many believe that parental consent initiatives are a central component of a broader conservative agenda to dictate, in federal and state law, the legal right of parents to control their children's upbringing—a right some allege has been largely usurped over the years by a wide range of governmental actions and programs.[37] Latinos, compared to other ethnic groups, have a more traditional value system with respect to sexuality.[38] (See discussion of *familism* and *respeto* in Chapter 2.) While the Latino culture emphasizes family and traditional values, it is important to enhance family communication skills about sexuality. Programs that aim to increase communication among Latino youth and their families must also work to empower individuals and communities. With the combination of traditional Latino cultural values and the conservative right's parental consent initiatives, the Latino community may be targeted with messages to deny teenagers' right to contraceptive services.

Recommendations

To ensure the continuation of confidential family planning services provided under Title X of the Public Health Service Act, the Child Welfare League of America and the National Council of Latino Executives recommend the following:

1. Encourage DHHS to solicit competitive proposals from family planning providers and others to serve the Latino community in a culturally appropriate manner. These proposals may include prevention, intervention, and outreach efforts that incorporate the world view and cultural values, attitudes, and norms of Latino adolescents. Cultural values of familism, mutual respect, and interpersonal relationships (*simpatica*) should be used to strengthen communication and relationship skills among Latino youths.

2. The President should submit FY 2000 budget proposal to Congress to increase Title X funding. Title X clinics should conduct vigorous outreach and assessment activities to assure the provision of culturally competent services to the Latino community. With the estimated 34% of Latino adolescents lacking health insurance, Title X clinics provide a entry to the health

care system. Additional funding and resources are needed for those clinics that provide services to the Latino community.

3. Health Maintenance Organizations (HMO) and other health insurers should provide comprehensive reproductive health services. Services should promote abstinence from sexual activity, as well as advocate for and provide appropriate medical services; i.e., a variety of health, education, and counseling services related to birth control, including contraceptive services, pregnancy testing and counseling, and information and referral.

4. DHHS and the states should develop aggressive strategies to educate Latino parents about sexuality issues. Several research studies identify the influence of Latino parents on their children. Employ Latino parents as peer educators to provide other adults in the community with the skills, information, and comfort level needed to reduce the risks of adolescent sexual behaviors.

5. DHHS and the states should increase efforts to inform the Latino community about youth's right to consent to family planning services and the importance of Title X. Outreach workers should be informed of Title X and its implication for the Latino community.

6. Undocumented aliens must have access to health care services. Community members should undertake aggressive outreach to provide information about services and to educate undocumented aliens as to their right and responsibility to obtain health care services. The services must be provided in locations that undocumented aliens perceive as safe havens.

7. DHHS should encourage states to conduct outreach to facilitate testing and treatment for Latino males under Title X. Programs should offer access to free or low-cost medical examinations, sexuality and male role counseling, and contraceptives.

8. DHHS and the states should conduct additional research in Latino male contraceptive knowledge, attitudes, and practices. Research findings should be widely distributed.

Notes

1   D. J. Landry & J. D. Forrest. (YEAR). How old are US fathers? *Family Planning Perspectives*, 27,159-161,165.

2   H. Miller, C. Miller, L. Kenney, & J. Clark. (1998). Issues in statutory rape law enforcement: The views of district attorneys in Kansas. *Family Planning Perspectives*, 30 (4), 177-181.

3   P. L. 104-193, Sec. 906.

4   Alan Guttmacher Institute. (1994). *Sex and America's teenagers.* New York: The Alan Guttmacher Institute.

5   L. Lindberg, F. Sorenstein, L Ku, & G. Martinez. (1997). Age difference between minors who give birth and their adult partners. *Family Planning Perspectives*, 29, 2.

6   E. Flores, S. Eyre, & S. Millstein. (February 1998). Sociocultural beliefs related to sex among Mexican American adolescents. *Hispanic Journal of Behavioral Sciences*, 20(1).

7   P. Donovan. (1997). Can statutory rape laws be effective in preventing adolescent pregnancy? *Family Planning Perspective*, 29 (1), 30-34.

8   Miller et al. 1998.

9   Donovan 1997.

10 Lindberg et al. 1997.

11 S. Ventura. (1997). *Births by age of mother by age of father, United States, 1995.* Washington, DC: National Center for Health Statistics.

12 United Nations. *Sexual and reproductive self-determination. State of the Work Population 1997,* Chapter 3. Available on-line at http://www.unfpa.org/swp97e/ch3.html#adolescent.

13 S. Elstein & N. Davis. (1997). Sexual relationships between adult males and young teen girls. Washington, DC: Author.

14 P.L. 104-194, Title IX, Sec. 912.

15 P.L. 104-194, Title IX, Sec. 912.

16 M. Kempner. (1998). 1997-98 Sexuality education controversies in the United States. *SIECUS Report*, 26, 6.

17 R. W. Blum & P. M. Rinehart. (1997). *Reducing the risk: Connections that make a difference in the lives of youth.* Minneapolis, MN: University of Minnesota, Division of General Pediatrics and Adolescent Health.

18 L. Kann, C. W. Warren, W. A. Harris, J. L. Collins, K. Douglas, B. Collins, B. Williamson, & L. J. Kolbe. (1996). *Youth risk behavior surveillance, 1995.* Atlanta, GA: Centers for Disease Control and Prevention, Surveillance and Evaluation Research Branch. As cited in E.M. Ozer, C. D. Brandis, S. G. Millstein, D. Knopf, & C. E. Irwin, Jr. (1998). *America's adolescents: Are they healthy?* San Francisco, CA : University of California, San Francisco, National Adolescent Health Information Center.

19 S. Davis & M. Harris. (1982). Sexual knowledge, sexual interests, and sources of sexual information of rural and urban adolescents from three cultures. *Adolescence, 17,* 471-492. As cited in L. M. Baumeister, E. Flores, & B. Marin. (1995). Sex information give to Latina Adolescents by parents. *Health Education Research,* 10(2), 233-239.

20 The Alan Guttmacher Institute 1994.

21 E. Flores. (1998). Latina Adolescent Pregnancy Prevention Symposium. New York

22 D. Kirby. (1997). *No easy answers: Research findings on programs to reduce teen pregnancy.* Summary. Washington, DC: The National Campaign to Prevent Teen Pregnancy.

23 Kempner 1998.

24 Davis and Harris 1982.

25 Centers for Disease Control and Prevention. (1991). Characteristics of parents who discuss AIDS with their children-United States 1989. *Mortality and Morbidity Weekly Reports, 40,* 789-791. As cited in Baumeister et al. 1995.

26 R. DuRant. (1990). Sexual behavior among Hispanic female adolescents in the United States. *Pediatrics, 85,* 1051-1058. As cited in Baumeister et al. 1995.

27 Sex Information and Education Council of the United States [SIECUS]. (1996). *Issues and answers: Sexuality education and the schools.* New York: Author.

28 A. Grunseit & S. Kippax. (1994). *Effects of sex education on young people's sexual behaviour.* Geneva, Switzerland: World Health Organization.

29 Pathfinders International. Involving parents in reproductive health education for youth. Available on-line at http://www.pathfind.org/PARENTS.html

30 Flores et al. 1998.

31 Flores et al. 1998.

32 National Family Planning and Reproductive Health Association. Facts about family planning. Available on-line at http://www.nfprha.org.

33 Alan Guttmacher Institute. Issues in Brief: Title X and the U.S. family planning effort. Available on-line at http://www.agi-usa.org/pubs/ib16/1b16.html.

34 Alan Guttmacher Institute 1994.

35 Alan Guttmacher Institute 1994.

36 Alan Guttmacher Institute 1994.

37 Alan Guttmacher Institute. Issues in Brief: Teenager's right to consent to reproductive health care. Available on-line at http://www.agi-usa.org/pubsib21.html.

38 Baumeister et al. 1995.

8.

Latino Adolescent Pregnancy Prevention

Central to the problem of early, unintended pregnancies among adolescents is the ability to make healthy decisions. Learning the values, skills, and goals for health decisionmaking is a lifelong task. It begins with healthy parents, and is reinforced by them throughout the child's life. But just as a child grows up in a family, parents and families exist in a larger world. We believe that families should have access to the support and the assistance of helpful community members and systems designed to their needs. These recommendations are ways that we can empower youth to be responsible about their sexuality and make healthy decisions about their sexual behavior, and how society can provide support to Latino families.

1. Adolescent pregnancy prevention programs must be aimed at primary prevention and address multiple factors.

Prevention requires a multipronged approach that addresses the capabilities, challenges, and potential of young people at each stage of life. No one program approach will be effective. Programs that address delaying sexual activity may be effective in reaching pre-adolescents and young adolescents. These programs should also include components to enhance communication about sexuality, relationships, and values between preadolescents and their parents or other significant adults, and opportunities to gain new skills. For middle adolescents, programs should promote assertiveness training and resistance skills, information on sexually transmitted diseases, encouragement of school achievement, and involvement in the community by participation in social, religious, cultural, volunteer, and recreational activities for teens ages 12 to 14. For older adolescents, programs should focus on setting goals, address sex role stereotyping as a potential limitation on their aspirations, provide strategies for avoiding unsafe sexual activity and skills for contraceptive access, and offer career planning and job exploration.

In addition, prevention initiatives should strengthen families, address other factors such as poverty and lack of opportunity, and provide educational enrichment and economic opportunities.

2. Develop programs that embrace the Latino culture and values. Programs should embrace family and cultural context of marriage, sexuality, and fertility.

The concept of culture is dynamic and ever changing. Many Latino adolescents participate in two cultures: the Latino culture of their parents and the culture of the wider community. Programs should build on Latino concepts of *familism* for adolescents to bring pride and honor to the family, *respeto* (respect), and *dignidad* (dignity).

Programs should be intergenerational and involve strategies that focus on groups of youth, neighborhoods, and families (rather than on individual behavior) and on parent sexuality education and parent-child communication.

Program components for effective programs should seek to reinforce clear cultural values and messages to strengthen group values and norms against unprotected sex.

Provide family counseling to address intergenerational conflict regarding changing gender role expectations within the context of family acculturation differences between parents and adolescents. Focus on helping the family to be flexible and to negotiate compromises and changes within the cultural value orientation. Reinforce same-sex relationships between parent and adolescents for information and support.[1]

3. Male involvement programs must focus on the needs and concerns of young men in the community beyond child support enforcement issues.

Programs for Latino young men should seek to provide healthy, positive male role models to assist boys in their identity struggle. Boys need to hear from male staff who can explore and express their feelings and who show a caring, vulnerable side. Programs should provide information on sex and sexuality to boys, improve communication between father and son and other adult males in the community, help boys to understand that there are consequences to risk-taking behaviors and to accept equal rights and responsibilities for their sexual decisions. Information on gender-specific attitudes, beliefs, and behaviors regarding romantic relationships, sexuality, and contraception must be included. Male involvement in casual, impulsive sex, and drinking must be included in program strategies. Linkages to educational and occupational opportunities for males must be explored.

4. Before developing a program, involve the community. Program developers should seek to become knowledgeable about the needs and characteristics of the community.

For organizations that are initiating a program in a Latino community for the first time, work with organizations already serving the Latino community. Share resources to expand program services.

Begin with a community advisory board to guide the development of the program until it is possible to build Latino representation in the organization's own board and staff. Hire residents to participate in the program in a variety of roles, including peer educators, community organizers, and administrators.

5. Involve adolescents in the development of adolescent pregnancy prevention programs.

Have youth identify the sociocultural issues impacting adolescent sexuality and participate in designing the programs to reduce risky sexual behavior. Peer health educators and peer leaders are just two ways in which youths can be involved.

Components for effective programs should involve group counseling that involve youth in small group exercises, which can

- provide basic information about risks of unprotected intercourse,

- provide basic information about strategies for avoiding unsafe sexual activity,

- address social pressures to be sexual,

- reinforce clear and appropriate cultural values and messages to strengthen group values and norms against unprotected sex,

- provide modeling and practice of communication and negotiation skills, and

- provide guidance for developing healthy relationships.[2]

6. Programs that aim to prevent adolescent pregnancy should provide educational enrichment and tutoring, as well as opportunities to increase the number of Latino adolescents who graduate from high school and enter college.

Several strategies are needed to reach Latino youth to assist them to complete high school. Traditional adolescent pregnancy prevention programs will not be as effective as programs that aim to increase life options. Any program that serves Latino youth must work to reduce the high incidence of early dropping out. Programs that emphasize career exploration and link job training and education have proven to be effective with African American youth. Similar programs must be developed and implemented in the Latino community.

7. Any Latino adolescent pregnancy prevention strategies must be family-centered and community-based with the goal to strengthen the family.

Programs aimed at reaching only Latino youth will not be as successful as family-centered programs. Programs must provide information and education to parents and community residents so that they have the skills, knowledge, and comfort level to discuss sexuality issues. Programs that include parents and community residents as the sexuality educators (who impart information and values within a Latino cultural context to their children) and that provide parents with opportunities for educational advancement are more effective in reaching Latino youth.

8. National and state adolescent pregnancy prevention organizations should be provided with information about Latino adolescent pregnancy prevention programs.

Programs may need to be retooled to address the cultural differences, influences, and impact on adolescent pregnancy prevention issues. Such programs should provide continuing education for professionals to give them skills to make assessments in culturally competent manner.

9. Funding communities need to increase their efforts to fund adolescent pregnancy prevention efforts in the Latino community. Model adolescent pregnancy prevention programs should be replicated across the Latino population and evaluated for effectiveness.

There is a lack of information of adolescent pregnancy prevention in the Latino community. Many adolescent pregnancy prevention programs have been evaluated for effectiveness and impact on
the white and African American community; however, little information is available regarding impact on the Latino community. In
addition, because of subgroup differences, programs must be replicated in the various subgroups.

**10. Improve data collection, analysis, and dissemination by
reviewing the current data and developing an action plan to
address the unidentified gaps.**

In developing this report, we were struck by the lack of data on
the Latino population. Only since 1989 have the states reported
Latino births to the National Center for Health Statistics. These data
have been helpful in the development of this report. We are concerned, however, that there is some movement away from the collection of data based on ethnicity. We would oppose any changes
that remove ethnic group delineation.

**11. Develop aggressive outreach programs targeted towards
adolescent Latino parents to ensure that they stay in school
or return to school after the birth of the baby.**

Provide intensive case management programs to link to services,
provide information on community resources, and monitor school at-
tendance and the school's response toward adolescent mothers. These
programs should also include education on parenting, child development, and careers, as well as information about higher education.

**12. Continue to have a dialogue with the Latino community
to tease out the relationship between traditional values and
adolescent reproductive health issues.**

The Latino community is not a heterogeneous community. Latinos of different national origins—Mexican American, Cuban, Do-

minican, Puerto Rican, individuals from Latin or Central America and others—are grouped together. Although they share a common language and heritage, there are differences among the many nationalities in cultural influences and histories. Discussions with the different subgroups around these issues should continue.

13. *Provide undocumented aliens with primary health care services that are specialized to meet their developmental needs.*

Communities should undertake aggressive outreach to provide information about services and to educate undocumented noncitizens or immigrants as to their right and responsibility to obtain health care services. The services must be provided in locations that undocumented noncitizens perceive as safe havens.

14. *Youths who are at high risk for pregnancy (out-of-home care, homeless, juvenile system) must be provided with human sexuality information, family planning services, and opportunities for educational and economic success.*

Human service providers serving Latino communities should provide comprehensive services that support youth development. Such programs should include educational and job opportunities, health care (including contraceptives for sexually active youths), outreach to parents to facilitate connection to community resources, parenting education, and life skills planning.

Topics should include but not be limited to discussions with caregivers on communicating about sex for early adolescents; resistance skills for mid-teens; and life options, career planning skills, and responsible decision-making skills about contraceptive use for older teens. Child welfare agencies should recognize that a history of child sexual abuse may be common among youth in out-of-home care. Sexuality education must include information on child sexual abuse. Family planning services should include a variety of health, educational, and counseling services related to birth control, including contraceptive services, pregnancy tests and counseling, and information and referral services. Life skills programs should include tutoring to improve school performance or provide employment training, role models, and mentors. These programs can assist youth in out-of-home care to understand the negative consequences of becoming parents and the impact of parenthood on their present and future plans.

States must develop and implement standards for comprehensive health services, including medical, nutritional, and psychological care for teens who are incarcerated or in out-of-home care.

Notes

1   E. Flores, S. Eyre, & S. Millstein. (February 1998). Sociocultural beliefs related to sex among Mexican American adolescents. *Hispanic Journal of Behavioral Sciences*, 20(1).

2   Flores et al. 1998.

9. Conclusion

Any effort to try to alleviate the problem of Latino teen pregnancy will require a sustained, coordinated commitment to a comprehensive, incremental, long-term program. There are no easy answers or quick fixes. Combating teen pregnancy must involve mobilization of an extraordinarily broad and diverse range of resources: families, religious groups, media, community and neighborhood groups, parent teacher organizations, the business community and labor, and public and private agencies in the areas of health, mental health, education, social services, income maintenance, and employment and training. Beyond increasing public awareness and mobilizing public and private resources, there obviously must be sustained and coordinated planning, program and policy development, service delivery, and monitoring.

Latino adolescent pregnancy is an issue that demands the leadership, the long-term commitment, and the courage to initiate the recommendations in this report. We have not definitively assessed the costs of such an effort, but we know that the price of even modest implementation of comprehensive prevention and supportive services will be high. The urgency of the problem of teen pregnancy in human terms compels us to move forward quickly and boldly.

Appendix A
Principles Underlying Program Development

1. Use a youth development approach.

The needs of young people must be the starting point for polices and programs. Provide the supports and opportunities that will best promote young people's competence and their connectedness to families and communities. Youth should be provided with the opportunity to act as mentors to young adolescents, peer counselors, and health educators in sexuality education programs.

2. Value individual strengths.

The program must build on the strengths of youth, their families, their cultures, and their communities. This begins with the recognition that every youth, every family, and every staff person has strengths. These strengths must not only be identified in service plans but must be clearly evidenced in steps for achieving goals.

3. Focus on the attainment of both tangible and intangible skills.

Intangible life skills such as decisionmaking, problem solving, critical thinking, self-control, and the assumption of responsibility for one's actions must be included as a component of adolescent pregnancy prevention programs. The concept of empowerment provides a useful lens through which to view service strategies that are youth driven. This concept implies that adolescents play a central role in case planning and the review of their own progress in decisionmaking about which services to use.

4. Learn by doing.

Values such as work ethics and attitudes cannot be learned through classroom-style teaching; they must be learned through active participation in work.

5. Recognize the roles of ethnicity and culture in program development.

Program must recognize and celebrate cultural differences and their importance to youth and their families. To enhance the ability of youth from racially and culturally diverse groups to access services effectively, agencies must employ bilingual staff and have access to resource materials and staff training on cultural issues that affect youth.

6. Promote open communication and responsible behavior.

The program must provide a safe environment for youth to openly ask questions about sex. This includes creating an environment that values individual differences and uniqueness, encouraging questions, and assisting youths to obtain information they cannot provide. The program should recognize that sexual relationships should never be exploitative and that premature sexual behavior poses risks.

7. Acknowledge gay, lesbian, and bisexual orientation.

An agency supportive of sexual minority youth must be staffed and administered by people who demonstrate a similar commitment to providing services that foster self-esteem and acceptance for gay, lesbian, and bisexual young people.

Appendix B
Focus Groups

Research with teens both sexually active and not sexually active should be an integral part of any pregnancy prevention efforts. Focus groups are one method of gaining qualitative information quickly and at a low cost. A focus group usually brings together between eight and 12 people to be interviewed by a trained moderator. Working with adolescents in a focus group on sexuality issues can sometimes be difficult because of the highly sensitive topic and adolescents' embarrassment, self-consciousness, and susceptibility to peer pressure. However, with a skilled moderator who can make the atmosphere feel safe and nonthreatening, an insightful and involved discussion among adolescent participants can occur.*

The following tool was developed with the end goal of involving Latino youth in the process of identifying issues, goals, and objectives for effective pregnancy prevention efforts in their communities. It is only a draft and may be modified to fit the reader's needs.

---

* W. DeJong & J. Winsten. (February 1998). *The Media and the message: Lessons learned from past public service campaigns.* CITY: The National Campaign to Prevent Teen Pregnancy.

Questions and Issues to Consider

Listed below are some questions and issues that need to be considered before conducting a focus group on adolescent sexuality and pregnancy prevention. The list of issues could be endless, but here we have provided a few of the main points to address when planning a focus group.

- What is the overall purpose of the focus group?

- What topics or areas do you want to focus on? This will determine the categories and questions. More questions that tap into prevention or intervention issues can be developed.

- Will this be a small focus group or a larger project? What is the scope?

- What age groups should you focus on? What regions or geographical areas should you focus on? For example, depending on the age group, you might want to ask questions about college or job training or questions specific to rural areas.

- You will need to develop a uniform set of protocols and format for conducting the focus groups. Who will be implementing the focus groups and where? How and from where will youth be recruited to participate? It may be easier for community-based programs to do the recruiting, because they have more direct access to youth.

- What resources will you need for the project, and where will they come from? Should you provide food for the group, and should you reimburse youth for their participation?

- What is the time frame for getting the project done? How will the focus groups be coordinated and by whom?

Background Information

1. Name: _____

2. Phone number: _____

3. Address: _____

4. Sex: ☐ Male ☐ Female

5. Age: _____

6. Are your natural parents ☐ Married ☐ Divorced

   ☐ Separated ☐ Widowed ☐ Living together

7. Who lives in your house? _____

   _____

8. Are you attending school at this time? ☐ Yes ☐ No

9. If yes, what grade are you in? _____

10. If no, what is the last grade you finished? _____

11. What racial/ethnic group do you identify yourself as? (Mexican, Puerto Rican ...) _____

12. Where were you born?

13. If not the United States, how many years have you lived in the United States? _____

14. Have you ever had sexual intercourse with a guy/girl?

    ☐ Yes ☐ No

15. For girls: Have you ever been pregnant? ☐ Yes ☐ No

16. For boys: Have you ever fathered a child? ☐ Yes ☐ No

Categories and Questions

Purpose of focus group

First of all, I'd like to explain the purpose of this discussion group. What we'll be discussing are your opinions about . . .

Information and communication about sex

Where do teenagers get their information about sex?

Who do boys talk to about sex?

Who do girls talk to about sex?

What kind of information do teenagers get about sex from their parents, friends, etc.? What does their mother/father/ best friend/boyfriend tell them about sex?

What makes it hard for parents to talk to their teenagers about sex?

Contraception

Where do teenagers get their information about contraception or birth control?

Who do boys talk to about contraception or birth control?

Who do girls talk to about contraception or birth control?

What kind of information do teenagers get about contraception or birth control?

Where do teenagers go to get contraception or birth control?

What makes it hard for teenagers to get contraception or birth control?

What makes it easy for teenagers to get contraception or birth control?

What makes it hard for teenagers to use contraception or birth control?

What makes it easy for teenagers to use contraception or birth control?

What methods of contraception or birth control do your friends or teenagers you know use?

Attitudes about sex

What are reasons to have sex?

What are reason not to have sex?

Why do your parents think you should not have sex?

Why do your friends think you should or should not have sex?

Why does your boyfriend/girlfriend that you should or should not have sex?

Attitudes about pregnancy

What are reasons to get pregnant or have a child?

What are reasons not to get pregnant or have a child?

Why do your parents think you should or should not get pregnant or have a child?

Why do your friends think you should or should not get pregnant or have a child?

Why does your boyfriend/girlfriend think you should or should not get pregnant or have a child?

Supports or resources for teen parents

What makes it hard to be a teen parent?

What makes it easier to be a teen parent?

What kind of support do teen mothers need?

What kind of support do teen fathers need?

Appendix C
Participants in the Latino Adolescent Pregnancy Symposium

The Child Welfare League of America and The National Council of Latino Executives would like to give thanks to all the attendees at the Symposium for their time, effort, hard work, and insight, without which this report would not have been possible.

Megan Annitto
3113 38th Street NW
Washington, DC 20016

Janice Bibb-Jones
NYS Office of Children & Family
    Services
40 North Pearl Street
Albany, NY 12243
Phone: 518/474-9461

Virginia Bishop-Townsend, M.D.,
    M.P.H.
Attending Pediatrician
Children's Memorial Hospital
2300 Children's Plaza, Box 16
Chicago, IL 60614
Phone: 773/880-3830
Fax: 773/281-4237
E-mail: v-bishoptownsend
    @nwu.edu

Gladys Carrion, Esq., Director
Inwood House
320 East 82nd Street
New York, NY 10028-4102
Phone: 212/861-4400
Fax: 212/535-3775

Wendy Castro
Program Coordinator, Adolescent
    Pregnancy
Child Welfare League of America
440 First Street NW, Third Floor
Washington, DC 20001
Phone: 202/662-4294
Fax: 202/638-4004
E-mail: wcastro@cwla.org

Debra Delgado, Senior Associate
Annie E. Casey Foundation
701 St. Paul Street
Baltimore, MD 21218
Phone: 410/223-2979
Fax: 410/547-6624
E-mail: debra@aecf.org

Maria Diaz, M.P.H., C.H.E.S.
U.S. Public Health Service
Office of Family Planning
26 Federal Plaza, Room 3337
New York, NY 10278
Phone: 212/264-5494
Fax: 212/264-9908
E-mail: mdiaz@hrsa.dhhs.gov

Samantha Figueroa
Program Coordinator
National Council of Latino
    Executives
Committee for Hispanic Children
    and Families
140 West 22nd Street, Suite 301
New York, NY 10011
Phone: 212/206-1090

Dr. Elena Flores
Department of Counseling
    Psychology
University of San Francisco
2130 Fulton Street
San Francisco, CA 94117
Phone: 415/422-6901
E-mail: florese@usfca.edu

Felix Gardon, Outreach Coordinator
Sex Information and Education
    Council of the United States
    (SIECUS)
130 W. 42nd Street, Suite 350
New York, NY 10036
Phone: 212/819-9770 x 311
Fax: 212/819-9776
E-mail: fgardon@siecus.org

Lupe Hittle, Director
Florence Crittenton Center
1105 28th St., P.O. Box 295
Sioux City, IA 51104
Phone: 712/255-4321
Fax: 712/2524743

Asari Innis
Former Program Coordinator
National Council of Latino
    Executives
Committee for Hispanic Children
    and Families
140 West 22nd Street, Suite 301
New York, NY 10011

Sarah Kovner
Special Assistant to the Secretary
U.S. Department of Health and
    Human Services
200 Independence Avenue SW,
    Room 605F
Washington, DC 20201
Phone: 202/690-6347
Fax: 202/690-7098

Bronwyn Mayden, Director
Florence Crittenton Division
Child Welfare League of America
440 First Street, NW, Third Floor
Washington, DC 20001
Phone: 202/942-0293
Fax: 202/638-4004
E-mail: bmayden@cwla.org

Luis Medina, Executive Director
St. Christopher's-Jennie Clarkson
  Child Care Services
71 South Broadway
Dobbs Ferry, NY 10522
Phone: 914/693-3030
Fax: 914/693-8325
E-mail: stchris_lmedina
  @hotmail.com

Maria Miramontes
Hablando Claro
Logan Heights Family Health
  Center
2204 National Ave.
San Diego, CA 92113
Phone: 619/685-1650 x 24
Fax: 619/232-7011

Elba Montalvo, President
National Council of Latino
  Executives
and Executive Director
Committee for Hispanic Children
  and Families
140 West 22nd Street, Suite 301
New York, NY 10011
Phone: 212/206-1090
Fax: 212/206-8093
E-mail: CHCFinc@aol.com

Aracely Panameno
Executive Director
National Latina Institute for
  Reproductive Health
1200 New York Avenue NW,
  Suite 300
Washington, DC 20005
Phone: 202/326-8970
Fax: 202/371-8112
E-mail: NLIRH@igc.apc.org

Karabelle Pizzigati, Director
Public Policy
Child Welfare League of America
440 First Street, NW, Third Floor
Washington, DC 20001
Phone: 202/942-0261
Fax: 202/638-4004
E-mail: kpizzi@cwla.org

Representative Alianza
  Dominicana
2410 Amsterdam Avenue,
  4th Floor
New York, NY 10033
Phone: 212/740-1960
Fax: 212/740-1967

Maria Rodriguez Immerman
Director
Casey Family Services -
  Bridgeport
2400 Main Street
Bridgeport, CT 06606-5323
Phone: 203/372-3722
Fax: 203/372-3558

Maria Rosado
Bureau of Children & Family
  Services
40 North Pearl Street
Albany, NY 12243
Phone: 518/474-9461

Joe Semedei
Committee for Hispanic Children
  and Families
140 West 22nd Street, Suite 301
New York, NY 10011
Phone: 212/206-1090
Fax: 212/206-8093
E-mail: CHCFinc@aol.com

Barbara Sugland, M.P.H., Sc.D.
Child Trends, Inc.
4301 Connecticut Avenue NW,
　Suite 100
Washington, DC 20008
Phone: 202/362-5580
Fax: 202/362-5533
E-mail: bsugland@childtrends.org

Catalina Vallejos Bartlett
National Latina Institute for
　Reproductive Health
1200 New York Avenue NW,
　Suite 206
Washington, DC 20005
Phone: 202/326-8970
Fax: 202/371-8112
E-mail: NLIRH@igc.apc.org

Robert "Bobby" Verdugo
Senior Fatherhood Parenting
　Facilitator
Bienvenidos Family Services
5233 E. Beverly Blvd.
East Los Angeles, CA 90022
Phone: 323/728-9577
Fax: 323/728-3483
E-mail: casinoble@aol.com

Dana Wilson, Director
Mid-Atlantic Region
Child Welfare League of America
440 First Street NW, Third Floor
Washington, DC 20001
Phone: 202/942-0288
Fax: 202/638-4004
E-mail: dwilson@cwla.org

Appendix D
Resources

General

Inwood House
320 East 82nd Street
New York, NY 10028-4102
Phone: 212/861-4400
Fax: 212/535-3775

Crittenton Center
P. O. Box 295
Sioux City, IA 51102
Phone: 712/255-4321
Fax: 712/252-4743

Casey Family Services - Bridgeport Division
789 Reservoir Avenue
Bridgeport, CT 06606
Phone: 203/372-3722
Fax: 203/372-3558

Committee for Hispanic Children & Families
140 West 22nd Street, Suite 301
New York, NY 10011
Phone: 212/206-1090
Fax: 212/206-8093

Curricula

Poder Latino: A Community Prevention Program for Inner-City Latino Youth
Available from Sociometrics
E-mail:
www.socio.com/program.htm
Community-based intervention targets Latino youth, ages 14 to 20, at elevated risk for HIV/AIDS. Works to increase awareness of HIV/AIDS by saturating target neighborhoods with public service announcements and encourages sexually active teens to use condoms.

Reduciendo el Riesgo
Education Training and Research Associates (ETR)
P.O. Box 1830
Santa Cruz, CA 95061-1830
Phone: 800/321-4407
Spanish language materials, including pamphlets on birth control, HIV/AIDS, puberty, STDs, abstinence, and monogamy. According to ETR, "Reduciendo el Riesgo/Reducing the Risk" has demonstrated

success in helping teens avoid unplanned pregnancy.

Como Planear Mi Vida
Advocates for Youth
1025 Vermont Avenue NW, Suite 200
Washington, DC 20005
Phone: 202/347-5700
Fax: 202/347-2263

Family Planning

Mary's Center for Maternal and Child Health
2333 Ontario Road NW
Washington, DC 20009
Contact: Elida Vargas
Phone: 202/483-8196
Fax: 202/797-2628

A bilingual health center for low-income, uninsured women and their children, primarily Latino. Offers culturally responsive services, including medical services, health education, and social services at the clinic. In addition, the clinic works with the schools through a Pregnancy Prevention and Health Education program.

White Memorial Medical Center Family Practice Residency Program
1720 Cesar Chavez
Los Angeles, CA 90033
Contact: Tina Tanner
MPH Program Administrator

This medical center has a health clinic that provides service to urban Latino youth ages 9-24. Services include primary health care, sexuality education, cultural awareness, contraceptive access and information, counseling, HIV/AIDS and STD prevention education, and referrals for a variety of other services to enhance the general well-being of adolescents.

Hispanic Health Council, Inc.
Program: Clinica Atabex
175 Main Street
Hartford, CT 06106
Contact: Elizabeth Delgado
Clinical Assistant/Health Educator
Phone: 860/527-0856
Fax: 860/724-0437

The Clinica Atabex of the Hispanic Health Council, Inc., is a reproductive health clinic for women and teens that offers free bilingual services: birth control counseling, free birth control, exams, and testing for pregnancy and STDs. The clinic is also beginning an outreach and educational program designed to raise awareness of teen pregnancy among Latino youth.

Infant Welfare Society of Chicago Adolescent Clinic
1931 North Halsted Street
Chicago, IL 60614
Contact: Susana Martinez
Phone: 312/751-2800

The adolescent clinic of the Infant Welfare Society offers pregnancy prevention services, including access to contraception, mentoring, counseling, sexual abuse assessment, and sexuality education. Delivery sites include a family planning clinic, home-based services, community agencies, and the Boys and Girls Club.

Guadelupe Center
2641 Belevue Street
Kansas City, MO 64108
Phone: 816/561-6885
Contact: Diane Rojas, Director

Mattie Rhodes Counseling and Arts Center
1740 Jefferson Street
Kansas City, MO 64108
Phone: 816/471-2536
Fax: 816/471-2561
Contact: Heather Dauzvardis
Program Director
The center provides services to girls ages 7-17. The Teen Group focuses on pregnancy prevention education and works to prevent early pregnancy among high-risk teens. All services are bilingual.

Casa Libertad
1905 Siringo Road
Santa Fe, New Mexico 87502
Contact: Jack Humphrey
Case Manager
Phone: 505/450-7991
An Independent Living Program that serves youth from different areas of the country (about 60% are Latino). Life Skills classes include contraception and counseling and also provide a nonjudgmental atmosphere for youth.

Parent Involvement

ASPIRA of Florida, Inc.
3650 N. Miami Avenue
Miami, FL 33127
Contact: Maria Teresa Jimenez
Phone: 305/246-1111

A pilot project in partnership with ASPIRA and the Office on Adolescent and Family Life. The target population is primarily migrant Latinos. The goal of the project is to reduce teen pregnancy by involving youth 9- to 14-years-old. The project promotes abstinence and provides intensive parent training.

El Lugar de Los Niños
Chicago, Illinois
This child care center was the first one to open in this Latino community of Chicago. The center works with parents as well as children to provide sex education.

Hablando Claro con Cariño y Respeto
Plain Talk Initiative Logan Heights
Family Health Center
San Diego, CA 92113
Contact: Marta Flores
Phone: 619/683-7563 x 145

Community

The Mexican American Services Agency, Inc.
130 North Jackson Avenue
San Jose, CA 95116
Phone: 408/928-1122
Fax: 408/928-1169
Programs specifically geared toward adolescent pregnancy prevention include Proyecto Acesso, a health education program, a male involvement program, and Familia Sana, which provides a holistic approach to preventing unwanted pregnancies and fatherlessness to adolescents and parents.

Support Our Students (SOS)
YMCA of Greater Winston Salem
Kernersville, NC
Contact: Carole Yardley
Executive Director
Phone: 336/722-9772
E-mail: sosymca@bellsouth.net

The "Amigos y Familia" program serves Latino students and their families in Forsyth County. Topics include responsible parenting, characteristics of an adolescent, an introduction to sex education, drug and alcohol abuse, and family communication with children.

School- and Community-Based Programming

La Casa de Esperanza, Inc.
Maternal Child Health Coalition
Prevention Group
410 Acadian Avenue
Wauhesha, WI 53186
Contact: Emilia Hernandez
Youth Program Coordinator

Program's goals are primary pregnancy and STD prevention for adolescents. The target population is Latino youth, including those in rural, urban, and suburban areas. The program is delivered at schools, neighborhood centers, places of worship, and community agencies. Information and services provided to teens include abstinence only, contraception information, STD education, substance abuse education, recreational activities, violence prevention, and vocational training.

Latino Youth 2000
La Alianza Hispana
409 Dudley Street
Roxbury, MA 02119
Contact: Diego Neira
Program Director
Maria Gomez, Outreach Worker
Phone: 617/427-7175
E-mail: Mullaney@meol.mass.edu

Latino Youth 2000 is a program of La Alianza Hispana. Services include contraceptive education and sexuality education, cultural awareness, tutoring services, HIV/AIDS and STD information, life skills, mentoring, peer education counseling, primary health care, and vocational training.

Mi Casa Resource Center
FENIX Program
571 Galapago Street
Denver, CO 80204
Contact: Barbara Bennett Rivera
FENIX Director
Phone: 303/405-4151

An HIV, STD, and teen pregnancy prevention program that uses trained teen peer educators to provide outreach and educational services for youth between the ages of 12 to 19. Peer educators from the target population are the key disseminators of the risk reduction services.

Male Involvement

Hablando Claro con Cariño y Respeto
Plain Talk Initiative Logan Heights
Family Health Center
San Diego, CA 92113

Contact: Marta Flores
Phone: 619/683-7563 x 145

The clinic makes significant efforts to include males in the design of the program, including Hablando Claro classes, training sessions, and community events. A male outreach worker serves to increase the number of male teens who use the services.

Always on Saturday
Hartford Family Action Plan
30 Arbor Street
Hartford, CT 06106
Contact: Flora Parisky
Chief Operating Officer
Phone: 860/232-0641

Part of a larger group of services called "Breaking the Cycle," which provides young males with the information they need to be sexually responsible and prevent pregnancy.

Hombres Jovenes con Palabra
15865-B Gale Avenue, Suite 1004
Hacienda Heights, CA 91745
Contact: Jerry Tello, Director
Phone: 818/333-5033

COMPASS
Adolescent Pregnancy Prevention, Inc.
1300 W. Lancaster Street
Fort Worth, TX 76102
Contact: Jeffrey Rodriguez
Phone: 817/338-4559

Program seeks to reduce adolescent parenthood among adolescent Latino males by discussing sexuality and encouraging positive behaviors such as completing high school and preventing gang membership. The program was designed specifically to reach Latino males. Places great emphasis on teaching that females are equals in relationships.

Mexican-American Community Center Services
130 North Jackson Avenue
San Jose, CA 95116
Contact: Enrique Arreola
Phone: 408/928-1122

Young Men's Clinic
Columbia University School of Public Health Center for Population and Family Health
60 Haven Avenue, B-3
New York, NY 10032
Contact: Bruce Armstrong
Clinic Coordinator

Abstinence Programs

PATH Program
Northridge Hospital Foundation
18300 Boscoe Boulevard
Northridge, CA 91328
Contact: Sandra Aldana
Phone: 818/901-4635

The "Pregnancy Abstinence for Pre-Teen Hispanics" (PATH) project is a prevention program for high-risk, primarily Hispanic youth. PATH uses trained peer-focused intervention targeting boys and girls in grades 5 through 8. After school workshops emphasize sexual abstinence and life and career options.

Southern California Youth and Family Center
101 N. La Brea, Suite 100

Inglewood, CA 90301
Contact: Annemarie Dalton
Phone: 310/671-1222 x120

A community organization that serves adolescents and families in the South Bay region of Los Angeles County. The Adolescent Abstinence-Based Learning and Education Project (AABLE) targets youth aged 9-14 years. The program also includes discussion with parents to develop strategies for communicating with their children.

El Futuro Es Nuestro
Lake County Health Department
3010 Grand Avenue
Waukegan, IL 60085
Contact: Pat Garrity
Phone: 847/360-2922

El Futuro Es Nuestro targets sixth-grade Latina girls attending Waukegan Middle Schools and offers primary prevention through small group activity sessions in the school. There are four main educational components: sexual health and drug and alcohol abuse education, development of goal achievement strategies, development of communication skills for parents, and mentoring for academic, career, and future family goals.

Watsonville YWCA
340 East Beach Street
Watsonville, CA 95076
Contact: Lorraine Phillips
Phone: 408/724-6078

A local, community-based agency in a rural community. The abstinence project targets two areas of the community that have been designated by the federal government as a Medically Underserved Population (MUP).

Vista Community Clinic
981 Vale Terrace
Vista, CA 92084
Contact: Fernando Sanudo
Phone: 760/631-5000 x1290

A private, nonprofit, community-based clinic that provides a wide array of health services. Offers an abstinence project for young adolescents and preadolescents in schools and community agencies in urban North San Diego County.

Mentoring

TEEN-Link Community Project YMCA
4776 El Cajon Boulevard, Suite 206
San Diego, CA 92105
Contacts: Rachel Humphreys and Guadalupe Meza
Phone: 619/229-9422

A prevention program that includes a Siblings/Friends Support Group, PRYDE after-school program, and Sibling/Friend Mentors. The PRYDE after-school program is offered to youth ages 9-14 who may be siblings and friends of pregnant and parenting teens, and, therefore, at higher risk of early pregnancy. The PRYDE curriculum teaches abstinence from sexual activity and about the health risks associated with adolescent sex.

National Organizations

Child Welfare League of America, Inc.
440 First Street NW, Third Floor
Washington, DC 20001-2085
Phone: 202/942-0293
Fax: 202/638-4004

National Council of Latino Executives
140 West 22nd Street, Suite 301
New York, NY 10011
Phone: 212/206-1090
Fax: 212/206-8093

National Center for Health Statistics (NCHS)
6526 Belcrest Road
Hyattsville, MD 20782

The National Coalition of Hispanic Health and Human Services Organizations (COSSMHO)
1501 16th Street NW
Washington, DC 20036
Phone: 202/797-4354
Fax: 202/797-4353
National Hispanic Prenatal Hotline: 800-504-7081

The National Council of La Raza
1111 19th Street, NW, Suite 1000
Washington, DC 20036
Phone 202/785-1670

National Latina Institute for Reproductive Health
1200 New York Avenue NW
Suite 300
Washington, DC 20005
Phone: 202/326-8970
Fax: 202/371-8112

Sexuality Information and Education Council of the United States (SIECUS)
130 West 42nd Street, Suite 350
New York, NY 10036
Phone: 212/819-9770
Fax: 212/819-9776

Annie E. Casey Foundation
701 St. Paul Street
Baltimore, MD 21202
Phone: 410/547-6600
Fax: 410/547-6624

For More Information

For more information, please contact

Bronwyn Mayden
Director, Florence Crittenton Division
Adolescent Pregnancy Prevention & Parenting
Child Welfare League of America
440 First Street NW, Third Floor
Washington, DC 20001-2085
Telephone: 202/942-0293
Fax: 202/638-2002
E-mail: bmayden@cwla.org